T0366580

Caring for Life

Diverse Economies and Livable Worlds

Series Editors: J. K. GIBSON-GRAHAM, MALIHA SAFRI, KEVIN ST. MARTIN, STEPHEN HEALY

Caring for Life

A Postdevelopment Politics of Infant Hygiene

KELLY DOMBROSKI

Diverse Economies and Livable Worlds

UNIVERSITY OF MINNESOTA PRESS

MINNEAPOLIS • LONDON

Portions of chapters 1 and 2 are adapted from "Multiplying Possibilities: A Postdevelopment Approach to Hygiene and Sanitation in Northwest China," *Asia Pacific Viewpoint* 56, no. 3 (2015): 321–34, doi.org/10.1111/apv.12078, copyright 2015 Victoria University of Wellington and Wiley Publishing Asia Pty Ltd. Portions of chapter 5 are adapted from "Hybrid Activist Collectives: Reframing Mothers' Environmental and Caring Labour," *International Journal of Sociology and Social Policy* 36, no. 9/10 (2016): 629–46, doi.org/10.1108/IJSSP-12-2015-0150; reprinted with permission of Emerald Publishing Limited; permission conveyed through Copyright Clearance Center Inc. Portions of chapter 5 are adapted from "Learning to Be Affected: Maternal Connection, Intuition and 'Elimination Communication,'" *Emotion, Space, and Society* 26 (2018): 72–79, doi.org/10.1016/j.emospa.2017.09.004, with permission from Elsevier.

Published by the University of Minnesota Press
111 Third Avenue South, Suite 290
Minneapolis, MN 55401-2520
http://www.upress.umn.edu

ISBN 978-0-8166-7985-0 (hc)
ISBN 978-1-5179-0160-8 (pb)

A Cataloging-in-Publication record for this book is available from the Library of Congress.

For Imogen

Contents

Introduction

There is no doubt that we need widespread social and economic change to avoid further environmental crises. Resource depletion, solid waste disposal problems, loss of biodiversity, climate disruption, and unequal access to the necessities and pleasures of human and nonhuman life are all directly related to the material objects and embodied habits of industrialized societies. In some parts of the world, waste management systems rely on large quantities of water and ever-increasing quantities of disposable hygiene products processed in overburdened landfills. Personal hygiene products with microplastic beads, beauty products with palm oil, and microfiber nappies shedding nonbiodegradable fibers through wastewater systems and beyond—these have all been implicated in a hygiene system that has vast distributed environmental effects on nonhuman life in oceans, rain forests, and atmospheres. However, at its heart, hygiene is not a set of material objects or chemical reactions. It is a social practice, embedded in many possible iterations of keeping health in different socioecological systems. This book dives deep into the everyday embodied hygiene and care practices of people caring for small children in two different parts of the globe, and examines how these practices connect with broader global transformations. Almost all of these people caring for small children are mothers; many of them are caring for grandchildren.

Why study mothers' caregiving when thinking about social change and hygiene? As a mother of four and a feminist geographer, I am aware of the dangers of focusing too much on the role of mothers in changing the world. After all, we have been blamed for everything from incel white supremacists to overpopulation to obesity. I am also well aware of the dangers of

placing our need for transformative change on the children of this genera-
tion, faced as they are with the overwhelming and anxiety-producing burden
of all the environmental and social sins of our forebears. Without discount-
ing the importance of all kinds of agents of transformative change, the
research for this book began with the everyday labor that mothers (in particular) are investing in the future of our shared world. I studied the everyday
labor of those caring for small children through place-based ethnographic
work in a multicultural urban center in northwest China and conducted
virtual ethnographic work with an online group of caregivers based mainly
in Australia and Aotearoa New Zealand. My work has been motivated by
my long engagement with development studies and environmental geography, as well as feminist political ecology and social studies of science and
technology. These fields, in various ways, are based on the consensus that
just knowing about and studying the effects of human activity does not
necessarily lead to future change. Investing in change is something that is
experimental, iterative, intentional, and tentative; it has no real guarantee
of success. Yet we attempt it anyway, for as Val Plumwood puts it, "If our
species does not survive the ecological crisis, it will probably be due to our
failure to imagine and work out new ways to live with the Earth, to rework
ourselves and our high energy, high-consumption, and hyper-instrumental
societies adaptively. . . . We will go onwards in a different mode of humanity,
or not at all."[1]
I have found it difficult to imagine alternative ways of living with the
Earth when it requires challenging and reworking my embodied habits.
Even when I become aware of the widespread ecological destruction that
certain hygiene habits might produce, the embodied nature of these habits
are so wrapped up in notions of disgust, the social expectations of others,
my everyday tasks and routines, and the norms of institutions around me
that it seems beyond my capabilities as an individual to rework them. The
consumer cultures I have grown up in have, over time, become reliant on
hygiene habits intertwined with consumer products. Aspects of this are now
being challenged, but the reliance on plastics, fragrances, foams, and animal
testing means that the ecological impact of our hygiene habits extends far
beyond the hygienic body in question. Likewise, the places I have grown
up with have complex water-based public sanitation infrastructures that
drain and mix all kinds of wastewater for chemical treatment and discharge.
Those wider hygiene systems are enforced not just by habits but also by
resource consent processes and industry norms, so they often seem too big

for the average person to influence. The materiality of hygiene in everyday life is so embedded, embodied, and habituated to all this that it is difficult to imagine and enact alternative ways of being together in the world—ways that are less resource intensive and waste producing. This is true to the degree that the hygiene habits and sanitation infrastructures of the Western world are still imagined as superior and are still exported to other parts of the world without much in the way of critical revision, where sanitation problems form part of an ongoing crisis emerging from urbanization.

Despite the seeming impossibility of meeting the challenge of reworking ourselves and our societies, many of us attempt it anyway. In order for widespread change to happen, we each need to be imagining and reworking ways to effect change in the spheres in which we find ourselves. Personally, much of my last seventeen years have been spent in the sphere of infant care and hygiene.

Anyone who has parented a child can tell you that infant care is an embodied and messy interpersonal practice that mixes the social and the material. Throughout the intense negotiations required as you attempt to care for a body other than your own, there are goals in mind: weaning and toilet training, both literally and metaphorically. Infants begin their lives completely dependent on their caregivers for both their input and their output, where sustenance and hygiene include actual food and waste as well as emotional and social regulation concerning what infants are exposed to and how they manage their reactions and make connections beyond themselves. Infants, we hope, end up as healthy young persons who can care for themselves in body, mind, and spirit and are able to care for others and places beyond themselves. The care practices we use to get them to such a state are complex, contingent, and diverse. They involve detailed negotiations over how to live together with others different from ourselves, how to manage power and knowledge differences, and how to remain cognizant of the needs and desires of multiple different stakeholders without forfeiting that future goal of healthy adult humans. What worked for some children, even in the same household, will not work for others. Even the most experienced parents must adapt and evolve with their individual children, situations, and the wider environment. There is no blueprint; there is no one right way, predictable outcome, or sure way to know whether the time and energy invested in particular practices are going to have the desired effect. Yet we continue to parent, care, invest, experiment, and hope, even if we end up accepting the blame for how our children turn out.

I will not write much more about parenting, but I hope you can see what I am trying to prefigure here. The task of reworking ourselves and our societies is something people are already doing. Caregivers of young children are already developing and reworking their embodied habits and those of their small charges, for better or worse. Although many of the ways we do hygiene are deeply embedded in habits that extend beyond rational decision-making, there are openings for change through negotiation and experimentation. It is possible to influence embodied habits and their connected social infrastructures. We may get it wrong, but it might be possible to influence change more broadly—and to influence change inside a time frame that can make a difference.

Two additional things have recently suggested the possibility of change. First, there is the way in which hygiene habits were deliberately—and in some cases drastically and rapidly—changed in the face of the Covid-19 pandemic. Although it was not easy, with the support of soft infrastructures, people all over the world reset their usual habits of handwashing, physical distancing, coughing and sneezing, face touching, and more. Just recently I listened to my son singing "Happy Birthday" to himself as he washed his hands in the bathroom nearby—this being the song he has been told comprises the requisite twenty seconds needed to kill the virus. Circles painted in picnic spots helped people stay far enough apart in San Francisco while dining outside. Duct-taped lines in supermarkets and coffee stands reminded customers where to stand while queuing. Masks were handed out as we boarded planes or entered university buildings. People commented that it felt weird to enter a building without sanitizing one's hands, donning a mask, or checking in via a contact-tracing app, or when someone offers a handshake rather than a nod. Many of us have become habituated to this new way of being together in public places—or indeed to our *not* being together in public places, drastically reducing travel for work and leisure, and reducing the spread of even normal winter illnesses. This was intended to be temporary, and in many places these precautions are lifting. The point is that change has been possible.

The second thing that suggests the possibility of change is the global diversity of hygiene practices. As I will argue in this book, hygiene is a place-based assemblage of practices. The places where I have conducted my empirical research into hygiene include a rather out-of-the-way part of China and a virtual place standing in for the Western world.[2] Qinghai province was the site of a year of ethnographic research in 2007 and three months of ethnographic research in 2009. I researched mothers' (including grand-mothers') everyday practices of care, paying particular attention to care work not usually counted as part of the economy. One of the most amazing care tasks I witnessed during this time was the practice of *baniao:* holding out babies to urinate rather than leaving them to do so in a nappy. Most babies were clothed in pants with a cutaway crotch, allowing this holding out to take place instantly and easily. I was fascinated. How was it possible to predict when a baby would need to eliminate, and to such a degree that nappies were not seemingly needed at all? What also struck me as interesting was the practice of bottle-feeding babies with formula milk was widespread, yet the practice of using disposable diapers or nappies did not make as much of a dent in traditional modes of nappy-free infant care. As I discuss later, both formula milk and disposable nappies seemed to have high levels of advertising, yet the globalization this represented was not occurring evenly in this out-of-the-way part of China.

My own sensibilities until that time had led me to believe that Westernization was occurring throughout the world and that multinational corporations were tweaking and even completely transforming diverse ways of being in the world through their nefarious advertising, lobbying, and social campaigns. Yet disposable nappies were not being taken up by all despite the huge amount of money invested in transforming nappy practices, particularly by disposable nappy producers Procter & Gamble. Indeed, I was not the first Westerner to be taken by this practice of infant toileting. I uncovered a whole network of people in Anglophone internet forums sharing their experiences adapting the practice to different contexts.

This puzzling experience diverted me—good ethnographic research is often diverting and diverted—into a whole new area of research where my thinking around postdevelopment and feminist geography was juxtaposed with the field of hygiene studies. What drove my interest was the way in which an intimate, embodied practice of infant care that required a large investment of time and energy seemed to have survived—and indeed thrived and spread internationally—in service to diverse values and ethics surrounding both baby and environmental health. To me, this had important implications for social change and different environmental futures. Other worlds are already present, and other worlds are already in the making. Maybe a different sort of global future is possible, especially if those of us in the Western world stop assuming our ways of doing things are the best and only ways. We can begin instead with an openness to other ways of being in the world that more adequately care for our commons. In one sense, then, this is a book about hygiene and infant care practices, but in another sense, at its heart, this is a book about the possibilities for change that are already here and already being enacted, which can be found if we are interested enough to look. The kind of change I am interested in is change that supports the flourishing of both human and nonhuman life. Like others, I have been interested in surviving well, survivance, flourishing, and more-than-human wellbeing,[3] but in this book, I have drawn inspiration from the phrase "guarding life."

GUARDING LIFE

The Chinese word for *hygiene* can be literally translated as "guarding life." As I discuss later, this translation comes from classical Chinese via Japanese and back; it is entwined in the histories of public health and modernization in Meiji-era Japan and the shifting power relationships between these two nations. Ruth Rogaski argues it is best translated as "hygienic modernity" because of the way it has been practiced as a modernization strategy. In China, Sean Hsiang-lin Lei returns to the original meaning in his historical work on hygiene assemblages in reformation-era China.[4] There is something beautiful in the notion of guarding life as a stand-in for hygiene. In much of the context of hygiene in public health and medicine, hygiene often draws more on ideas of killing germs than guarding life. Although the war on germs has reemerged in some parts of the world in response to Covid-19, the notion of being kind has been the driving response in my own country, Aotearoa New Zealand. Guarding life and being kind draw on our collective ties, our desire for communal wellbeing, and our ability to work together to protect the lives of the most vulnerable among us. In this hygiene assemblage, disinfectant and sanitizer worked alongside social practices of care. For me, this involved isolating in our home for four full weeks in one of the world's strictest lockdown responses, which garnered widespread support from all over the country.[5] "Be kind, stay home" is the message we were invited to respond to while we waited for the virus to be eliminated from our islands or for a vaccine to be invented, with government-issued payments that made isolation possible for those whose work could not be carried out from home. Although this is not a book about New Zealand's response to pandemic, recent events have highlighted how important it is to pay attention to the full extent of a hygiene assemblage, including the social and economic elements, if we are serious about widespread change.

What do I mean by a hygiene assemblage, and why is it an important concept? I mean here the materialities, socialities, and spatialities of hygiene that we see gathered in particular places at particular times. These materialities, socialities, and spatialities are culturally situated. They can draw from quite different cosmologies (understandings of the universe), ontologies (understandings of what is real), epistemologies (understandings of how we can know what it is we think we know), and methodologies (ways of finding things out). The hygiene assemblages I discuss in this book are place-based assemblages drawn from different understandings of the world. I have drawn on Chinese assemblages of hygiene, or *weisheng,* a word comprising the ideographic characters for "guard" and "life." Such assemblages of hygiene are not fixed in place but can travel and shift through time and space. They can be tweaked to provide better chances of guarding life too, but only if we pay attention to the particularities of what is being assembled, where, and how and why it is assembled in such a way.

Changes in hygiene and sanitation are often understood to be part of "development," a nebulous industry, practice, and worldview exemplified in global organizations like the United Nations and the World Bank. However, as will become clear, my understanding of hygiene change resists such simplistic notions of goal setting and technical transfers of knowledge. Too often these kinds of approaches to change reproduce and replicate problematic norms from resource-intensive parts of the world, with little understanding of what they replace. I am more interested in a postdevelopment approach to hygiene and guarding life. Such an approach would start with deep understanding and appreciation for the particular and diverse hygiene assemblages already present in different parts of the world. Such places are usually seen as places to be "done to" in terms of hygiene, rather than to be learned from.

As such, a postdevelopment approach to guarding life is political. It seeks to decolonize hygiene in such a way that people in the minority world stop assuming their situated hygiene assemblages are the best and will work evenly everywhere in the majority world in much the same way. The minority world here refers not to a particular place on a map of low- and high-income countries; it is not a stand-in for notions like the developed world, the first world, or the West. Rather, the minority world is the world in which reside a minority of the world's population by accident of birth—the diplomats and CEOs of Javanese Indonesian society, the broad swath of supposedly middle-class Americans, and, of course, the global cosmopolitan elite with their hotel franchises and fluffy white towels that look much the same in Suzhou, Tokyo, San Francisco, and Lagos. Minority world is shorthand for those who do not live in the majority world—the underside of Beijing migrant worker communities with no formal residency or rights, the self-organized slum communities of Jakarta and Dhaka, Indigenous Australians living in rural isolation without access to midwifery or general practitioner services, refugees in vast tent cities on the borderlands of Kenya, and ordinary subsistence farming folk in the rural parts of the planet, living life as their ancestors had. The majority world inhabits realities distinct from those of the engineers who have imagined sanitation and hygiene to be primarily about water, and the doctors and nurses and public health workers who have imagined hygiene and sanitation to be primarily about education and individual behavior. As will become clear in the remainder of this book, the hygiene practices of the minority, Western world should not just be exported wholesale and intact to every part of the world.

Indeed, it seems that minority world hygiene practices do not work well even in the minority world. Even wealthy parts of the United States faced a breakdown in health care and government as Covid-19 ravaged the nation. But it is not just the United States, whose health care system is notoriously expensive and ineffective; the United Kingdom and Sweden have also faced health system overload. We are finding everywhere in the world that hygiene is a practice embedded in the politics and particularities of place. The sanitation systems that support hygiene practices in the minority world are resource intensive and built for a time when water resources and the ocean seemed vast and infinite. What is required is not a general roll-it-out approach to hygiene but rather a slow, listening approach, one responsive to place and aware of the broader assemblage of which hygiene is just a part. In other words, what is required is the same kind of attentive approach we might take in raising a child, but on a much broader scale. Indeed, as a species, we need to listen and respond to our environment; we need to learn to be affected by the world around us and to appropriately rework our practices of health keeping, economy, and domesticity. Those of us in the minority world need new hygienes and new modernities. We need to learn how to live better with each other and with the more-than-human world. We need different kinds of hygiene systems, and we need to start with as broad a range of possibilities and knowledges as is feasible.

A postdevelopment politics of hygiene is one that deconstructs the assumptions of development, displacing the idea that the rich countries of the minority world know more about modern hygiene and sanitation. A postdevelopment politics of hygiene replaces this idea with an attentiveness to the multiple hygiene modernities keeping health globally and to the embodied politics of change that might enable majority world modernities to assist transitions to sustainability in the minority world. The prefix *post-* in postdevelopment invites thinkers to move beyond the restricting categories and colonial presumptions undergirding the development project and to instead identify the multiple political moves that have violently imposed development in neocolonial projects—as well as to think through how an embodied politics of place might produce something else. As I have written elsewhere, a postdevelopment approach must start where we are and then multiply possibilities, thereby increasing our options for transformation and transition to different kinds of hygienes and different kinds of modernities better attuned to the nuances of ecosystems in place as well as to the Earth's broader systems.[6] A postdevelopment approach to hygiene change does this in such a way as to move hygiene assemblages toward those that guard life in all its complex, interconnected magnificence.

A POSTDEVELOPMENT POLITICS OF HYGIENE

Hygiene change is political. It involves power and decision-making. I have already proposed that a postdevelopment politics of hygiene must start with an attentiveness to the nuances of specific hygienes in place. As a researcher, I developed this attentiveness as I worked to document the diverse hygiene practices of an out-of-the-way part of China using in-person ethnographic methods. I researched hygiene in place in the city of Xining, in Qinghai province, for over three years (Figure 1). It is not a minority world place, despite China's economic growth over the last thirty years, but rather part of the majority world. It is a place where development is imposed by outsiders through demolition and construction projects. At the time I was conducting my research, I had my oldest child with me, who was four months old during the first scoping trip in 2006, a toddler during the one-year ethnographic trip, and three years old in the last major interviewing trip in 2009. It seemed a good idea to participate in local practices of infant hygiene as a way to partially embody the care practices of the people I was researching. This practice in turn led me to another community of interest.

As part of learning how to do nappy-free infant hygiene, I joined the forum OzNappyfree, an online group hosted by Yahoo! Groups, which at

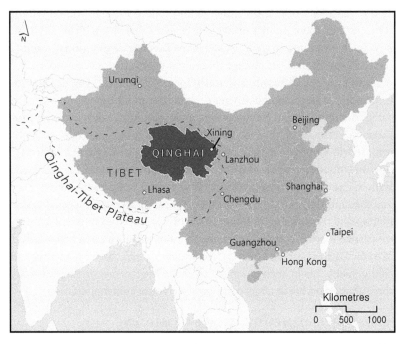

FIGURE 1. Map showing location of Xining and Qinghai within the region. Map by Nina Muijsson, 2022.

the time comprised some four hundred parents based in Australia or New Zealand seeking to learn and discuss practices of infant toileting known variously as nappy-free hygiene, natural infant hygiene, or elimination communication.[7] This group had splintered from a global group dominated by American mothers some years before, mainly because the antipodean participants had realized that hygiene was indeed situated in place and culture. It quickly became clear that this group was informing my research in deeply meaningful and interesting ways as they sought to learn from practices in the majority world, including grilling me repeatedly on how things worked in China's far west. I adapted my research accordingly,[8] and in 2009, I collected a full year of posts from this group. In 2010, I analyzed them for insight into how the practice was adapted in these specific Western countries. I have published some of these insights,[9] but over the years I have had many requests for something that more substantively described and developed this work. I did some follow-up research with the group in 2015 and stayed in contact with the various Facebook offshoot groups that followed as online forums declined in popularity.

Throughout my time researching and writing this book, I wrote and archived a variety of short ethnographic and autoethnographic descriptions and reflections from the three different countries where I spent time. I extended these reflections as I had more children and found myself situated in different hygiene assemblages. I began writing about these assemblages in 2007 with my first toddler, and I completed these in 2020 with my fourth toddler. Some of these reflections appear as interludes between chapters, their purpose being to evoke the feeling of being in place before the more academic analysis takes over. Readers can use these as a way to reorient themselves to other perspectives. They break open the black box of academic research, exposing the highly situated assemblages and reflections of this body, doing this research, in this particular place and time. As such, they also serve as a feminist and decolonial practice of situating knowledge by bringing attention to the politics and mechanics of knowledge creation—in this case, by a Pākehā (New Zealand European) mother of four, an academic, and a fieldwork researcher. Each interlude shows me differently positioned with respect to city and country of residence, employment, study, and parenting situation and support, and this makes a difference.

Knowledge is certainly situated; these embodied ethnographic interludes communicate that this book is both about understanding some of these situated hygiene assemblages in out-of-the-way places and about inspiring and enacting social change in a damaged and broken world. This book, then, is the beginning of a postdevelopment politics of hygiene, where good change is not something dished out from the developed world to the developing world (or the modern to the backward). In chapter 1, I lay out the argument for such a postdevelopment politics based on guarding life rather than merely killing germs or rolling out homogeneous sanitation infrastructures. Using the work of a variety of postdevelopment and poststructural theorists, I make the case for thick and rich descriptions of diverse hygiene, mothering, and care practices as a first step in marshaling possibilities for needed change in both minority and majority worlds. I propose hygiene assemblages as a way of researching and representing hygiene in its multiplicity, across multiple cultures and knowledges and places. An interlude invites readers to enter the hygiene assemblage in western China, as I did as a young mother being schooled by grandmothers in infant care. In chapter 2, I turn to a thick description of the practice of baniao as a mode of infant toileting as it is practiced and assembled in the city of Xining, in China's western region. I begin to map out the assemblage of hygiene in western China by beginning with this practice before moving outward to examine other strands of the assemblage that enable it. These other strands include the limited uptake of disposable nappies in the early 2000s, as well as the understanding of children's bottoms as *tai nen*—very delicate— for reasons that draw on traditional Chinese medicine understandings of bodies, qi, blood, and health. An interlude follows recounting an interview with a maternity nurse who switches between biomedicine and traditional Chinese medicine as she discusses her role teaching others to breastfeed and her own journey as breastfeeding person.

In chapter 3, I delve deeper into traditional Chinese medicine and the history of hygiene in China in order to think about the way assemblages shift and move over time between multiple ontologies of the body and health. I describe the medical and healing traditions that inform how care-givers and mothers in China understand their own bodies and the bodies of their infants. I examine the historical intersections of Western and Chinese medicine and discuss the hybrid forms that emerged via the friction of awkward engagements (to adopt Anna Tsing's language). An interlude follows introducing the kinds of bodies and spaces of infant hygiene I experienced as I moved from China to Australia to New Zealand with subsequent children.

Chapter 4 launches into a thick description of the hybrid hygiene practices of Australian and New Zealand practitioners in what is known as elimination communication (EC), following the practice from birth to toileting maturity as represented in the OzNappyfree Yahoo! web forum. The hygiene practice draws on Chinese practices and understandings of infant hygiene but adapts them for a Western culture and spatiality. I examine this as a postdevelopment project of knowledge exchange in which the knowledges and norms of majority world places such as Xining are understood as having value for urban Australia and New Zealand in the minority world. While this chapter examines the way EC works in households as practiced mainly by mothers, I connect the practice to the wider hygiene assemblage emerging from the OzNappyfree forum. The OzNappyfree forum, however, had more intentionality than a basic assemblage, and in chapter 5, I advance the argument that the forum can be understood as a hybrid collective experimenting with change. The hybrid collective pushes the practice of EC from the nuclear and atomized domestic practices of individuals or nuclear families and into a broader social collective that has the potential to inspire more widespread changes in hygiene practices in the minority world.

Finally, in the short, concluding chapter 6, I ask how all of this might constitute a postdevelopment politics of hygiene that works across multiple places to guard life in all its forms, both human and more than human, in minority and majority worlds. I put forward a vision of a pluriversal politics that eschews the Great Singularity or the one-world world. Such a politics actively engages with assemblages in place to see diversity in terms of both practice and ontology. Such a politics works to multiply possibilities rather than force a singular vision into reality. Such a politics seeks to nurture our capabilities for "being together in place"[10] for the health of our bodies, our communities, and our planet.

This book is about the possibilities for good changes that are collectively, tentatively, and experimentally developed in multiple places through stories and practices, and the politics of direct action and proliferation that bring some of these possibilities to life. The effects of changing one or two hygiene practices spark changes further afield, including social norms, infrastructures of care, and wider knowledge commons. Direct hygiene action is not just about the individual people or households that begin it but is also about the broader community that might take up such changes as they become further normalized and supporting. We all start life in the home, and proliferating changes in the home and everyday practices can spark broader material and environmental change. It is the presence of these multiple (and potentially ubiquitous) hygienic modernities, multiple possible might-have-been and could-be histories and futures, that allows a politics of real social, economic, and environmental change to flourish. This is what J. K. Gibson-Graham refer to as a politics of possibilities: an uncertain, hopeful, experimental postdevelopment agenda that challenges us to imagine and practice development and hygiene differently, to make other worlds possible—perhaps even the dignified worlds Roelvink speaks of.[11] We can shift hygiene assemblages, but we need to do much more. This book shows how it is crucial to incorporate attentive consideration of embodied knowledges and habits into postdevelopment approaches, particularly when thinking and enacting the "different mode of humanity" that Plumwood calls for. It is with this in mind that I proffer *Caring for Life* as a rallying point for rethinking and reassembling not just hygiene but also social change more generally in these troubling times.

1 Thinking Multiplicity

> Our thinking needs to be in the service of life—and so does our language. This means giving up preconceptions, and instead listening to the world. This means giving up delusions of mastery and control, and instead seeing the world as uncertain and unfolding.
>
> —Scholars Concerned for Life in the Anthropocene,
> *Manifesto for Living in the Anthropocene*

> A process of reworlding . . . doesn't try to smother differences. [It is] one that envisions a "pluriverse" rather than a universe, welcoming heterogeneity rather than enforcing a singularity.
>
> —Ruha Benjamin, *Viral Justice*

Right now seems like a bad time to publish a book challenging hygiene norms in the minority world. With the Covid-19 pandemic, observing excellent hand hygiene and disinfecting all surfaces with germ-killing substances are no longer primarily the preserve of those employed in the health care industry or those with obsessive-compulsive anxiety. Given this context, I should clarify now that by approaching hygiene in a critical way, I will not be arguing that hygiene is purely a cultural construct. I will, however, be arguing for multiplicity when it comes to thinking about hygiene because hygiene, like any practice, is deeply situated in place. Places are multiple and diverse, so hygiene is too.

This means that now is an excellent time to be writing and thinking about hygiene multiplicity. By multiplicity, I attempt to name and grasp something that is at once intuitive and counterintuitive: we seem to live in a series of interacting but multiple realities that are culturally situated, place based, and ontologically distinct. These realities do not exist in isolated bubbles. Rather, they travel, interact, dominate, disappear, and reappear; they may even form hybrids. Realities are produced culturally, but they also have materiality, temporality, structure, and substance. Even in a global pandemic, hygiene realities only partially overlap, producing cognitive dissonance in places where conflicting realities clash. Sanitation and hygiene projects in the majority world are fraught with development and cultural assumptions about bodily norms and infrastructure, both now and historically. There is much to be learned from attending to multiplicity in hygiene—and in development.

In this chapter, I develop a framework for multiplying possibilities through the work of postdevelopment theorists who critique one-size-fits-all development. I put this into conversation with assemblage thinking to develop a concept of hygiene assemblages. However, I do not leave these hygiene assemblages disconnected from history or power struggles. In the world of the development industry, sanitation and hygiene are treated as universals. Knowledges are developed in the developed world to be exported (or educated, or exemplified) to the developing world. A postdevelopment critique of hygiene and sanitation programs problematizes the ways that Western notions of health and hygiene—and Western infrastructures of hygiene—are assumed to be the best and most appropriate in any situation, with this particular knowledge assemblage thought to be more real than any other hygiene realities or constructs already in place. These assumptions are problematic on a number of levels, including the perspectives of efficiency, appropriateness, wellbeing, and possibility. Instead of viewing hygiene and sanitation as universal, I propose that we consider hygiene as an assemblage—that is, as a suite of practices, materials, infrastructures, biota, and more that somehow cohere to keep health.[1] I provide examples of situated hygiene assemblages that look different from universalist notions of hygiene that usually emerge in development projects, arguing that postdevelopment approaches to hygiene must start in place with what is already keeping health. These embedded hygiene assemblages in place are thus best understood as multiple realities, interacting with other realities that partially overlap and are shifting fractally.

What does this approach to multiplicity mean when moving forward with postdevelopment approaches to hygiene? Intentionally working to think multiplicity is the only way I can move forward in studying hygiene and health-keeping practices in the far west of China, where the realities of infant and maternal bodies only partially intersect with my own. The work of thinking multiplicity is never done. Just when you think you are able to fully grasp, engage, and inhabit multiple realities, a previously unrecognized universal might arrive on the scene, and the work begins again. I finish with some methodological reflections on researching in and with diverse bodies across multiple places, and on how sketching the constitution of these hygiene assemblages requires an embodied approach to thinking and knowledge making.

RETHINKING HYGIENE

Hygiene and sanitation development projects are based around the hygiene practices of the Western world, which have been developed through particular interactions with particular places, as I will explore in this chapter. The statistics tracking the achievement of the global sustainable development goals, for example, specifically exclude collectively owned and public toilet facilities from sanitation indicators,[2] and they tend to link concerns about hygiene with those of water under the acronym WASH (water, sanitation, and hygiene). But could the semiprivatized hygiene arrangements favored by the Western world be harmful for people and the planet? In contemporary times, Sarah Jewitt argues that indeed they are, and from both environmental and social justice perspectives. In her article "Geographies of Shit," she problematizes the "Northern" preference for expensive and wasteful flush toilets along with water-based sanitation systems, which are not necessarily any more effective in terms of hygiene or smell than ecologically friendly dry systems. All over the world, entrenched cultural norms, neocolonial development structures, powerful emotions, and deeply embedded taboos around human feces combine with "a lack of academic curiosity" to create barriers to thinking up alternative "excreta management systems."[3]

In her work, Jewitt is particularly concerned with the infrastructure of sanitation systems—those large-scale, (mostly) water-based public works that are the quintessential marker of hygienic modernity. When she refers to alternative "excreta management systems," she is mostly referring to alternatives to these public water-based systems found in developing countries. But perhaps "alternative" is not a helpful way of considering the matter; it labels whatever is outside the water-based systems as other and minor in comparison. Indeed, in places such as China, a diversity of management systems exist and partially overlap, even in cities.[4] Many of these systems function well and may be useful for consideration by the developed world. For example, Shervin Hashemi has researched the sustainability of two systems in Korea: septic tanks (water-based systems) and more traditional resource-oriented sanitation systems, where human waste is envisioned as a source of nutrients rather than only as a waste product.[5] Hashemi found that the latter resource-oriented system is effective and sustainable by both community and sanitary indicators, including water usage. Deljana Iossifova's work in China problematizes the shift to water-based sanitation systems.[6] She notes both the loss of nutrients from rural farms resulting from the disruption of traditional service-networked sanitation systems, where night soil workers remove waste from homes or central transfer stations and deliver it to rural areas for conversion to fertilizer. The disruption of such systems has resulted in an increase in open defecation as cities in China struggle to provide water-based sanitation systems for everyone.

This is not to say that there is no need for wellbeing and community projects focused on improving hygiene and sanitation. While both Jewitt and Iossifova are critical of water-based sanitation systems, they also recognize that the wrap-and-toss system of excreta disposal used in toiletless households in the Global South is deeply problematic.[7] Jewitt points out that wrapping feces in plastic bags and tossing it out in a variety of inappropriate places leads to water contamination problems, not to mention plastic pollution. But inappropriate sanitation is not limited to the Global South. Currently the infant excreta management system used for the vast majority of Australian babies is not too dissimilar from a wrap-and-toss approach.[8]

Although disposable nappy companies recommend that caregivers flush feces before disposing of the nappy, the practice is certainly not widespread, with most of it being wrapped in the nappy and tossed out in household rubbish collection bins, ending up in landfills. According to the *Guardian*, a single baby in the Western world may get through four thousand to six thousand nappies in their nappy career. A total of 167 billion disposable nappies are produced each year, using 248.5 million barrels of crude oil.[9] Most end up in landfill—or worse, dumped inappropriately. While not entirely like the wrap-and-toss system Jewitt describes, it is also a less-than-ideal way to dispose of fecal matter; it is wrapped up in a protective shell and cannot easily break down, and neither can the paper and plastic comprising a disposable nappy. Some estimates say it could take five hundred years! Given that more than 300,000 disposable nappies are used per minute, the problem seems too big to even begin addressing. Yet some countries have. Vanuatu has moved to limit the use of disposable nappies after decades of pollution and contamination,[10] and Western countries have struggled to address environmentally problematic infant hygiene practices. Jewitt notes that the "deeply embedded taboos surrounding human feces have often . . . created barriers to the development of more effective and / or sustainable excreta-management systems."[11] This is true in places with all kinds of sanitation systems and infrastructure, and no less so in the minority world.

Forms of hygiene that require more (or different kinds of) bodily contact with human waste are often viewed with disgust by those habituated to water-based, sit-down toilet systems,[12] and are taboo or completely off the table for discussion in development planning and sanitation engineering design. These taboos around systems of sanitation and practices of hygiene become problematic when environmentally damaging systems spread to become the norm at a large scale. This is not to say that running water is not an important public provision; it is. But running water is a separate thing from solid waste management, and sanitation systems are entangled with embodied hygiene habits. Given the concerns for social justice in hygiene expressed by writers like Jewitt, the sustainable development goals aimed at increasing access to affordable sanitation, as well as widespread concerns about the ecological footprint of the minority world, the time is certainly ripe to openly consider different kinds of hygiene practices. It is important to make sure, however, that the way we do this is not more of the same old colonizing "one true hygiene" approach to health. This requires situating particular domestic hygiene practices within broader contexts of knowledge, science, society, economy, culture, health, and place. It requires understanding how such practices are constituted by and woven through multiple lived experiences. What works in Vanuatu may be different from what works in rural Ukraine or urban Kenya or coastal New Zealand, and within these places, what works may be different for different kinds of bodies, family living arrangements, and age groups. Hygiene, after all, is an assemblage of spatialities, socialities, and materialities.

I now turn from sanitation systems and infrastructure to look in more detail at the kinds of domestic hygiene practices that reflect and are influenced by these broader social and material systems. These domestic practices can be significant in their potential to influence and change, tweak, and twist the broader reality in ways we might not fully appreciate. As bodies change their habits, wider social norms and infrastructural materialities may also change. Hygiene facts may start to change because hygiene evidence in science is often built on cultural assumptions around hygiene and the body—embodied norms that start from practices in the home. I will develop this idea further throughout the book, but for now, I point out that studying hygiene from the view of domestic and personal practices is still unusual, despite the role personal hygiene plays in embodied geography and in geographies of the body.[13] Some of this reluctance to delve into domestic hygiene practices is probably the result of the distaste that academics (and others!) exhibit for the details of sanitation—what has sometimes been identified as a masculinist distaste that extends to the abject, leaky, messy bodies represented in the domestic spaces of hygiene.[14] Perhaps the relative mundaneness of personal and family hygiene has obscured it from academic study for so long; historical records of state health interventions are far more common than those dealing with the day-to-day management of personal hygiene. Our own practices of personal hygiene have been habituated and embodied to the point of becoming almost invisible (and unquestionable), which can prevent researchers from exploring it further.

One researcher who has influenced thinking about hygiene as a practice is Elizabeth Shove. Shove's work on cleanliness, comfort, and convenience provides important insights into how the bodily habits of people in the minority world both form and are formed by the indoor infrastructure of bathrooms and running water. Expectations for cleanliness were heightened as personal hygiene infrastructure changed; this consequently shifted notions of what was required to be an accepted member of society in terms of the cleanliness of clothing, the frequency of showers, and so on. Shove's most influential work in practice theory is of relevance here: she draws our attention to the formation of regimes of comfort and cleanliness and "how meanings, practices and technologies hold together" and thus "influence the rate and direction of change."[15] Her work presents deeply textured evidence from the minority world suggesting that changes in the environmental impact of hygiene are related to both global-scale processes of technology change and embodied habits and practices influenced by social and cultural expectations. She points out the contingency of things that may have been taken for granted as unavoidable: bathroom use could have been otherwise (and indeed was), and laundry practices and expectations can be different. Paradoxically, increasing reliance on convenience devices has resulted in further fragmenting of activity, "inadvertently exacerbating the sense of harriedness and generating demand for yet more convenient solutions."[16] We could say this has been associated with sociotemporal re-structuring in the Global North. I will return to this point later as I exam-ine the different temporalities of caring for infants in different parts of the world and what this enables in terms of hygiene practices. Shove's ongo-ing work has examined the intersections of domestic practices, consumer technologies, and social and environmental change, pushing against behav-ioralist approaches that frame social change as related primarily to atti-tudes and choices.[17] Shove's work has implications for my project in that her conceptualization of change makes space for critical analyses of hygiene assemblages in place without dismissing the possibility of intentional change in the interests of people and planet.

From what has been discussed so far, it seems clear that some forms of hygiene might be harmful to the environment, so it may be tempting to think about hygiene and place in terms of trade-offs between human well-being and environmental wellbeing. However, inappropriate hygiene prac-tices introduced from elsewhere can also have human costs. This was first brought home to me in an interview with an observant community pedia-trician and development worker in rural Qinghai, the province in north-west China where I conducted fieldwork. She told me of the many cases of cold damage she saw in her ten years of maternal and child health work with nomadic and farming communities. Women showed her their bent and stiff fingers, damaged by frostbite, frostnip, or other nonfreezing cold injuries. Although cases of cold damage are obviously not unknown in this harsh, high-altitude environment, its relative frequency on women's hands was attributed by this doctor to an astonishing source: the seemingly innocuous practice of handwashing. A staple of health education projects on the plateau, recent decades had seen the promotion of frequent hand-washing and its subsequent adoption by many nomadic and settled Tibetan communities. Despite the apparent increase in cases of cold damage, this has generally been celebrated as a health achievement.

Keeping hygiene through handwashing after every toilet stop and animal-related task is a given for health and development professionals in both China and the industrialized Western world. Health experts and develop-ment practitioners may assume that handwashing is a universal truth of good hygiene rather than a practice that has developed within particular contexts of health keeping and disease transmission. Because developing countries are often conflated into a single category on the basis of a limited number of economic and health indicators, health practitioners may over-look the variety of disease vectors within this diversity of disparate places. A typical statement runs as follows:

> The two biggest killers of children in the developing world today are diar-rheal disease and respiratory tract infections. The simple act of washing hands with soap can cut diarrhea risk by almost half, and respiratory tract infection by a third. This makes handwashing a better option for disease prevention than any single vaccine. If developing countries are to achieve their 2015 mil-lennium development targets for reductions in child mortality, this unfin-ished agenda of the 20th century must be completed. Not only must water and sanitation become universal, but so must the habit of handwashing with soap.[18]

From this starting point, the thinking of development, health, and gov-ernment workers often goes as follows. The Qinghai–Tibet Plateau is not a wealthy or developed place, and certainly it has high child mortal-ity.[19] Therefore, the above statement applies, and the best solution is to run a handwashing promotion program. Teaching assumed-to-be-ignorant Tibetan women to wash their hands with soap and water is assumed to be crucial to improving health outcomes in the region.

Yet the barren and cold high-altitude plateau is a place with its own spe-cific health dangers. Water on the hands at temperatures of −30°C is not a hygienic practice, if we take the *Oxford English Dictionary*'s definition of hygiene as "practices or conditions conducive to keeping health," or the traditional Chinese definition of "guarding life."[20] This fact is recognized in the health advice provided to Western travelers to the plateau, who are warned to use alternative sanitary measures to manage the microbes that contribute to disease because of the danger handwashing poses in terms of cold damage and frostbite.[21]

For much of recorded history, handwashing has been common practice before eating all over the world,[22] including in nomadic Tibet, where hands, not utensils, are used to eat traditional foods. However, the scientific fact of frequent handwashing as a means for disease prevention is based on disease transmission vectors for specific diseases (especially those between animals and humans) in settled societies. Historically and today, it is the sedentary, agriculturalist societies with more crowded living conditions, altered ecosystems, and more intensive agricultural practices that have witnessed the development of animal-to-human infectious diseases.[23] New diseases—many of which were unknown to Indigenous, hunter-gatherer, nomadic, or more isolated societies all over the world—have tended to originate in these (often developed) places, such as the heartland of Chinese civilization and vast areas of Europe.[24] Although Tibetan communities have a variety of agricultural practices that could also contribute to these sorts of diseases, my point is that hygiene practices develop in particular settings in response to particular disease trajectories, particular microbial communities, and particular risks to health.

Drawing on Shove's understanding of social practices, then, we can imagine hygiene practices such as handwashing to be a particular set of practices and understandings situated within a wider network of practices, materialities, and understandings that we call hygiene. This wider network includes economic, environmental, social, medical, cultural, and political particularities. It includes the material conditions currently present or manifestly absent: water, oil, soap, bacteria, worms, microbes, dirt, blood, feces, animals, doctors, snow, wind, ice, jackets, fire, stoves, and fuel. It also includes the meanings assigned to all these things. Understanding handwashing in this way works to make visible the often overlooked linkages between disease and context, to make present that which was previously absent and silent. Handwashing in Tibet is handwashing that occurs in a different reality from those imagined by development workers and hygiene enthusiasts from the minority world.

In the West, the hygiene practice of frequent handwashing is less situated in the historical trajectory of disease development and more rooted in the historical trajectory of obstetric intervention.[25] In the late nineteenth century in the Western world, women began giving birth in hospitals in increasing numbers. Here they were under the supervision of doctors and obstetricians—usually professional men with multiple patients in the ward—rather than traditional midwives or family general practitioners who visited them in their homes. In hospitals, they faced increased risk of cross-contamination and puerperal or childbirth fever as a result of the vaginal examinations performed by obstetricians moving between patients and even from autopsies to patients, transferring infection as they went. The immediate health risks of a particular cohort (people giving birth) in a particular space (the hospital obstetric ward) at a particular time (the mid-1800s) gave rise to a hygiene practice (handwashing) that responded directly to these risks—as well as having far-reaching implications for other diseases. However, on the Qinghai–Tibet Plateau, health risks are of a very different sort than those in the heartland of China or in nineteenth-century hospitals. Tibetan hygiene practice development had been situated firmly in the context of coping with a harsh, cold climate, especially among nomads. Historically, nomads on the plateau have avoided washing with water, instead using butter or oil to protect their skin against the drying effects of the wind, sun, and cold. How can these traditional knowledges be incorporated into hygiene practices on the contemporary plateau?

Handwashing is, without a doubt, an important strategy in preventing the ingestion of the potentially fatal hydatid worm, especially for people who frequently interact with dogs and sheep.[26] Still, from the prepandemic perspective of someone living on the plateau, the longer-term threat of hydatids or the intangible concern of influenza or diarrhea played against the shorter-term realities of cold damage—and for many, it was rational to first avoid cold damage. This rational decision is sometimes interpreted by authorities as another example of the supposed irrational, backward thinking of the Tibetan people, or their preference for dirtiness. Academics and development practitioners may presume a lack of knowledge of correct hygiene practices and seek to teach correct behavior.[27] In doing so, however, they are essentially following the behavioral approach that Shove critiques as unrealistic and ineffective in initiating change while perpetuating neocolonial stereotypes that value globalized expert-generated facts over situated, place-specific knowledge. The point here is that hygiene is situated in place and time, and its particular practices are likewise situated within broad networks that lack direct causal paths. Although we can trace the practice of handwashing back to hospitals and obstetric developments, this path was not inevitable because we can likewise trace Tibetan hygiene practices back to particular historical and environmental trajectories and situations. Studying the ways that these different hygiene practices and understandings develop, clash, interact, and are gathered anew reveals to us the situatedness of our own embodied and habituated hygienes. We may thus begin to perceive what makes certain practices appear as common sense and others as nonsense. What seems like nonsense may in fact make more sense as we struggle to rework and situate hygienes that are responsive to changing environments, economies, and communities of people, animals, and microbes.

In the case of handwashing on the Qinghai–Tibet Plateau, it is doubtful whether these handwashing projects have helped with hydatid transmission, as Bai and colleagues found that the chance of contracting hydatids was not related to education level or even necessarily dog ownership, but to sheep ownership and hunting.[28] Yet the recent Covid-19 pandemic doubtless means that handwashing may once again become more important than avoiding cold damage, especially for those traveling further afield—although this is not necessarily always the case. If would-be modernizers on the plateau could put aside the feelings of disgust or dismay that less regular handwashing regimes may provoke, they might facilitate other solutions that protect the hands of Tibetan women from cold damage and the livers of their families from hydatid-induced cysts.

What this story reveals is the value of thinking and critique outside the assumptions of development. My approach to thinking about economic and geographical differences in hygiene is informed by postdevelopment critical theory. I find that postdevelopment thinkers challenge my deeply held assumptions about the nature of reality, although they are sometimes critiqued for their lack of solutions. In the next section, after I provide an overview of postdevelopment thinking, I will use it to develop an approach to studying hygiene multiplicity across geographical and cultural diversity.

POSTDEVELOPMENT AND THINKING MULTIPLICITY

In light of the above reflections on handwashing on the Qinghai–Tibet Plateau, it is clearly problematic to impose one form of hygiene across diverse places. Hygiene has often been associated with modernity, and modernity in turn has been associated with development. For much of its intellectual and practical history, the goal of development has been to transition societies and economies from traditional to modern. The dawn of the development era is often traced to U.S. president Harry S. Truman's (in)famous inauguration speech calling for America to lead "a bold new program," sharing its scientific advances with the world. Since that time, the concept has been built on teleological language that assumes the path of modernization taken by the industrialized Western world is universal and inevitable, while also paradoxically taking great effort on the part of would-be developers.[29] Postdevelopment scholars, like postcolonial scholars, have sought to disrupt Eurocentric norms and show how the transition to homogeneous modernity is neither inevitable nor universal; rather, it is built on a violent, racist erasure of economies, societies, and cultures.[30] The *post-* in postdevelopment thus implies development is under the microscope, permitting analysis of a world in which the idea and practice of development has been deeply intertwined with colonialism.[31] Elise Klein and Carlos Eduardo Morreo, in their 2019 book *Postdevelopment in Practice*, provide an overview of postdevelopment thinking. They note that postdevelopment scholars have consistently shown how development's models of progress normalize individuals over collectives and capitalist economies over other forms of economy. They also note how postdevelopment scholars have identified powerful Eurocentric discourses in development that privilege Western expertise and systematically overlook and devalue traditional knowledges and social systems.[32] In the same volume, postdevelopment scholars Esteva and Escobar, reflecting on twenty-five years' worth of postdevelopment scholarship, point out that development cooperation under the World Bank and mainstream NGOs might lead to "some improvements for some people" but overall reinforces colonialist understandings of development and thus normalizes dispossession as modernization.[33]

In much the same way, current global development initiatives such as the United Nations' sustainable development goals enact what John Law has called a "one-world world."[34] These initiatives assume that all the world's varying and diverse places are small subgroups of an overarching reality. Each of these different places is represented by statistics and indicators that frame the world as a collection of relatively homogeneous individuals and processes. Development is understood as the movement of more and more of these places into statistical profiles that look more and more like those of OECD countries. Development thinking often works to erase possibility by enacting a teleological view of reality where everyone in the world performs a version of modernity that includes broadband internet, flush toilets, and equal numbers of women and men represented in a parliamentary democracy. In more liberal understandings of development, there is recognition that cultural differences might mean modernities look slightly different when it comes to the details of voting processes, toilet design, and smartphone uptake, but the understanding often remains the same: these cultural differences are merely preferences, perspectives on a single reality.[35] This view is not without critique. Indigenous scholars in particular have long critiqued this "one-world world" view of reality, as have scholars from the majority world. Since the ontological turn, many other minority-world scholars have also recognized the multiple ontologies in which we all participate.[36]

In this vein, scholars from a variety of places have traced and researched other modernities, by which I mean the differential ways in which people and places have both resisted and accommodated supposedly inevitable universalizing forces.[37] These other modernities may not look like what is often meant by the term *modernity* in the popular sense. Whether in out-of-the-way places such as Indonesian rain forests[38] or Tibetan hospitals,[39] or in higher-profile places such as the East Asian Tiger nations or China's southern industrialized cities,[40] these modernities have interacted differently with various global trajectories and processes, resulting in different contemporaneous realities. I deliberately emphasize "contemporaneous" because I refuse to organize people and places into some kind of "historical queue," where some are behind but destined to follow the same problematic path of industrialization and modernization as those who are ahead.[41] The so-called behind or backward places are just as much the result of contemporaneous global interactions and interconnections. Their different economies and societies are not in the past but in the present; they are contemporaneous. This is not to say we should romanticize all places and ignore issues of global inequality in power relations. Rather, it is to say that processes of (neo)colonialism, extraction, exclusion, and more produce interconnected modernities. All these diverse, interconnected places in the world are modern—differently modern, but in this line of thinking, modern nonetheless. It seems to me that the arranging of places into a historical queue is a way that linear thinkers trapped in a one-world world seek to reconcile the rich and incredible global diversity of place, economy, environment, and culture.

Currently, in the social sciences and humanities, it is relatively easy to garner acceptance for the idea of other modernities, particularly the idea that these modernities are interrelated and coproduced rather than somehow behind.[42] But it has been less common to read these other modernities as sources of hope and of alternative futures for our shared Earth, although postdevelopment writers from the Global South have been arguing this point for some time now. For example, Escobar wonders at the "tremendous inability on the part of Eurocentric thinkers to imagine a world without and beyond modernity," arguing that in this world of multiple modernities, it is not acceptable to think of a Western modernity as the Great Singularity.[43] Escobar's work has focused on translocalisms, where trajectories of change are multiple and located and can lead to multiple future local and global states. He calls this multiplicity a pluriverse.[44] Likewise, other postcolonial scholars reject the "monoculture" of modernity and try instead to make visible an "ecology" of economic and social practices, or other modernities. They ask us to focus on emergences and to inquire into already emerging alternatives because they are already on the "horizon of concrete possibilities."[45] A growing number of authors are highlighting these emergences as a form of postdevelopment social change or a pluriversal politics of sustainability.[46]

In this book, I join these postdevelopment authors in a bid to move away from a monocultural conception of a single possible modernity to ecologies or multiplicities of contemporaneous modernities that allow unexpected hybrid varieties to flourish. For me, the commitment to thinking multiplicity is an ethical one that starts from a recognition that much of the world's troubles come when one group of people impose their vision or version of reality on other groups. There is a danger for people like me who want to see a different world; we run the risk of blinding ourselves to the many worlds that already exist and are perhaps already modeling the changes we seek. It is in interacting and overlapping diverse economies, ecologies, and realities that creativity and adaptation can lead to glimpses of both beauty and survival. I like to think of the Earth as a series of diverse, fascinating, beautiful, harsh ecosystems—multiple interlocuting realities—that have held together, survived, and sometimes flourished. It is when a particular way of being in the world is developed and universalized as the only reality that we end up in messes like anthropogenic climate disruption, biodiversity crashes, and microplastic-infused melancholia.

What would it look like to explore an international ecology of interrelated hygiene modernities? How does the emergence of the unexpected hybrid variety of infant hygiene I describe later in the book fit into these multiple realities and possibilities? My view is that by focusing on these emergences in hygiene, we can better imagine future hygiene modernities that better care for our bodies and our environments. In what follows, I argue that in paying attention to diverse hygiene modernities, we might find the resources to remake minority-world relationships with their environments already present and available—in terms of an embodied hygiene relationship, and potentially spilling over into other areas of our societies and economies. As has become clear in the global response and fallout of the Covid-19 pandemic and its associated economic shutdowns, our bodies, and thus our health, are intimately linked with both economies and modernities. Our hygiene measures are embodied, are embedded in place, and have impacts beyond our individual households. Our diverse measures for guarding life through hygiene practices are at once minutely intimate and expansively global. Diversity and multiplicity are concepts that have implications for hygiene practice and challenge one-world notions of reality in fundamentally transformative ways.

THINKING MULTIPLICITY IN HYGIENE STUDIES

The problem of thinking multiplicity is not only a central concern for postdevelopment thinkers describing pluriverses. It is also a central concern of new materialism and assemblage theory, where writers like Donna Haraway, Maria Puig de la Bellacasa, Annemarie Mol, and Bruno Latour critique social theorists for continuously invoking and reifying preexisting social structures in explaining social phenomena. For scholars influenced by this body of theory, such social structures are not taken for granted or inevitably reproduced by immovable power relations. Instead, they are created, recreated, and sometimes entrenched through specific assemblages of things and their social relationships in specific times and places.[47] Assemblage thinking allows us to be specific about how things are held together and to imagine a reassembling that is not necessarily absorbed in reproducing dominant structures, even if it is possible that this might happen. Katharine McKinnon uses assemblage thinking to sidestep combative approaches in the birthing room to "ask how what we come to call patriarchy is being enacted through the complex networks that coalesce in the birthing room,"[48] and thus how it might be reworked into something else. She catalogs a multiplicity of diverse actants, including objects and discourses, attempting to "untangle how each of the actants make certain actions possible . . . to formulate different kinds of engagement [that] calls us to a different sort of engagement, collective rather than combative."[49] Thinking about multiplicity through new materialism and assemblage theory allows a different kind of possibilist engagement: guarding life through health care, and allowing, for example, the recognition of multiple ontologies of the body to be acknowledged in improving health outcomes in places as diverse as Laos, China, Australia and New Zealand, and the Pacific.[50]

Annemarie Mol's work has brought us the idea that reality—including material bodies and their illnesses—is enacted. In *The Body Multiple,* she reminds us of Latour and Woolgar's work, which shows how science constructs reality materially in the lab by uncovering and interpreting traces of new substances. She reminds us of Judith Butler's careful work on how gendered realities are performed into existence, even in material bodies.[51] However, Mol asks us to consider that "maintaining the identity of objects requires a continuing effort." She intentionally drops the word "performativity" in order to use the verb "enact," highlighting the "complex present" in which the identities of objects "are fragile and may differ between sites."[52] She goes on to note that "if an object is real, it is partly because of practice. It is a reality enacted."[53] This is important for my thinking about hygiene and about fieldwork. We are first freed from the idea that we must uncover the right reality and the accompanying anxiety that arises when what we uncover is different from other people's ethnographic work. More importantly, however, we might come to see how change happens in and through performance and enactment. Different realities come into play partly depending on what we—researchers and writers—are paying attention to. I will return to this point later.

Mol's thinking on multiplicity is, like mine, grounded in her ethnographic fieldwork. In her study of the biomedical condition of lower-limb atherosclerosis, she asks what exactly atherosclerosis is. The answer is complex, she discovers, and multiple. The consulting room, the therapy room, microscopy, the operating room, the radiology department, the ultrasound suite—each space and method describes atherosclerosis differently. Sometimes these differing descriptions come together in a single patient: pain while walking, results of clinical examination and/or angiography, surgical intervention, and pathology may all somehow fit together to produce a single coordinated atherosclerosis. More often, however, the relevant practitioners find themselves faced with "poorly coordinated realities," where contradictions occur between the results of pathology and the life of the patient, or between angiography and other instruments. There are rules of thumb for discriminating between contradictory versions of atherosclerotic reality—for deciding, in fact, what reality is. Frequent contradictions require the frequent application of these rules of arbitration. We can see then that these poorly coordinated realities are not definite and fixed in form but vague, fluid, indefinite, connected, and enacted. Mol writes:

> In a single medical building there are many different atheroscleroses. And yet the building isn't divided into wings with doors that never get opened. The different forms of knowledge aren't divided into paradigms that are closed off from one another. It is one of the great miracles of hospital life: there are different atheroscleroses in the hospital but despite the differences

between them they are connected. *The body multiple* is not fragmented. Even
if it is multiple, it also hangs together.[54]

As will become apparent later in this book, the idea of the "body multiple" has underpinned my thinking around hygiene, infant bodies, and the
maternal and caregiving bodies that support them. What this adds to the
pluriversal and multiple modernities approach of thinking about multiplicity is an ability to think multiplicity within a single body. It is relatively
easy to think of multiple ontologies when they conveniently stay fixed in
different parts of the world, where their cosmologies, histories, and lan-
guages are distinct both geographically and conceptually. But how do we
think about multiplicity when it is right here in front of us, as it is when
development practitioners travel, or when researchers conduct fieldwork
somewhere far from their home countries, or when two cultures of work or
medicine meet in a single workplace? How do we think about multiplicity
when two different ontologies of the body meet, as is the case when the
understandings of the body conceptualized in traditional Chinese medicine meet those of the biomedical sciences in a single person? It is here that
Mol's conceptualization of the body multiple helps us think about multiplicity in nuanced ways. It is particularly helpful in thinking about the birthing, breastfeeding, and caregiving bodies and subjects that emerge between
traditional Chinese medicine and biomedicine in the interviews and ethnography to come. I am not alone in finding this way of thinking helpful,
as attested by the growing new materialist theoretical engagement in the
field of hygiene studies in East Asia and beyond.

The field I am calling hygiene studies is not a recognized discipline as
such. However, there does exist a disparate collection of English-language
publications by scholars from the fields of science studies and medical history who have taken it upon themselves to link projects of hygiene to issues
of power, colonialism, development, and modernity in a usefully critical
way. The key text in the area is Ruth Rogaski's book *Hygienic Modernity:
Meanings of Health and Disease in Treaty-Port China,* which is a masterful
history of the concept of the Chinese word *weisheng* and its connections
with the treaty port city of Tianjin, and with modernity in China more
generally.[55] Sean Hsiang-lin Lei published his modern history of Chinese
medicine in 2014, *Neither Donkey nor Horse: Medicine in the Struggle over China's
Modernity,* which draws on a number of key pieces of research adopting a
new materialist take on the history of hygiene in China.[56] As will become

evident in chapter 3, both these histories have been deeply influential for me, as have the works by a cluster of scholars researching histories of hygiene and hygiene modernities in an East Asian historical context, evidencing some influence from science and technology studies.[57] Other resources include *East Asia Science, Technology, and Society (EASTS)*, a journal at the cutting edge of postcolonial and feminist science and technology studies, including important work on hygiene. I have also connected with researchers associated with the Sustainable Infrastructure project, who have published work in critical hygiene and sanitation studies of urban China and India. Their work is based on the everyday hygiene practices of local people rather than large-scale engineering projects assuming compliance with the hygiene and sanitation directives of public health experts.[58]

Outside East Asia, other major publications in the field include Virginia Smith's history of personal hygiene; Mary Douglas's anthropological study of the concepts of purity and taboo; an edited collection on geographies of dirt; explorations of the biological aspects of hygiene and disgust; feminist geographers' contributions to studies of the body and its fluids; and a number of journal articles and book chapters that deal directly with global diversity in hygiene.[59] There is also an extremely large, but less relevant, body of medical, health, and development studies literature that takes hygiene or sanitation as its subject.[60] However, it does so in a nonreflexive, uncritical way, assuming that hygiene is a Great Singularity progressively revealed to the world as science and biomedicine advance understanding and practice along the path of one true hygiene.

In recent times, microbial scientists have started to question the conflation of hygiene with a reduction in bacteria or virus load (that is, killing germs), given the large quantity of emerging literature on the importance of our microbiome.[61] This helps many recognize some of the value of different and traditional practices of hygiene, diet, and approaches to cleanliness.[62] Yet the goal so far has been to redefine hygiene universally and then make plans for its (even more consistent) implementation in research and public health—that is, to require further reeducation of those still embroiled in traditional practice. While the recognition that hygiene should be about more than killing germs is certainly an important step, I am not interested in this type of engagement with hygiene. My concern is that this type of engagement still smacks of colonialism, where the norms of the West are often subconsciously performed as normal through scientific health research, shown through well-funded studies to be valid, and then applied uncritically to the rest of the world as best practice. Scientific studies are important, and there is no criticism here of scientists trying to improve understanding within their fields. What I am saying is that there is a role for thinking about the knowledge production process, which can unintentionally reproduce false hierarchies of practice and knowledge, as we will see later in this book in the area of infant toilet training research.

In contrast, a postdevelopment politics of hygiene must be acutely aware of the power dynamics of knowledge production, especially as it affects the wellbeing of people both near and far from centers of scientific and medical research. A postdevelopment politics of hygiene is one in which the everyday practices and norms of people in out-of-the-way places are first assumed to be highly adapted to their place and environment. A postdevelopment politics of hygiene must be decolonizing; it must challenge the implicit assumptions underlying health care and research, which normalize white and Western bodies and cultures and problematize all others. It requires moving away from the Great Singularity of one true hygiene toward situated hygiene practices, with overlapping realities that are multiple and contemporaneous. Given this review of multiplicity in hygiene studies, it seems time to lay out the approach I take to thinking about hygiene across culture, space, and time.

HYGIENE ASSEMBLAGES

Hygiene, in both English and Chinese linguistic traditions, originally referred to an array of health-keeping practices, mainly those that people could implement themselves.[63] However, people do not make decisions around health-keeping practices alone; they do so within a range of culturally, socially, and even politically prescribed options, in a particular place and specific environment. In light of my earlier discussion about hygiene on the Qinghai–Tibet Plateau and the dangers of isolating hygiene practices from place, it makes sense to conceptualize our situated hygiene as an assemblage. A hygiene assemblage can be situated in a specific place yet still be interwoven with international flows and influences. This is the conceptual framework I use to approach hygiene in the remainder of this book.

My understanding of assemblage has been influenced by John Law's treatment of method, where he uses the term *method assemblage* to refer to both methods and the extended circumstances and knowledges implicated in methods—what he calls the "fluidities, leakages and entanglements that make up the hinterland of research."[64] In the same way, we can conceptualize a hygiene assemblage that refers more broadly to the bundle of practices, materialities, socialities, spatialities, subjectivities, and entanglements that make up the hinterlands of hygiene and are themselves implicated in, and produced by, hygiene practices and beliefs. In the case of hygiene, this includes embodied practices of health keeping, such as washing, sterilizing, and mask wearing; the materialities of practices surrounding water, chemicals, and bodies; the socialities of these material practices, such as caregiving and shame, class and empire; the spatialities of sociomaterial practices such as clean and dirty spaces and the relationships between them; the travels of health extension workers and Daoist sages; and the subjectivities (or senses of self) that are formed and tied up in all this in and through place and practice. I imagine these assemblages to form and reform in the present but to also be a "simultaneity of stories-so-far," where multiplicity is not just multiplicity in space but also in space-time.[65] Thus, the histories of hygiene, along with their multiple temporal and spatial trajectories, form part of the current assemblage of hygiene in place.

Why use "hygiene assemblages" rather than "hygiene practices" or just "hygiene"? I sympathize with readers rolling their eyes at such affectations of language, but the term *hygiene assemblages* allows us to signal a departure from the monocultural, monospatial fixed rules of hygiene as they are imagined in Western medicine and most development literature. This does not devolve into a kind of "strong constructionism," where the stretch and travel of knowledge—and of science in particular—is entirely dismissed.[66] To appropriate John Law's words, hygiene is thus explicitly situated in a broader bundling or recursive self-assembling assemblage

> in which the elements put together are not fixed in shape, do not belong to a larger pre-given list but are constructed at least in part as they are entangled together. This means that there can be no fixed formula or general rules for determining good and bad bundles, and that . . . [the assemblage] grows out of but also *creates* its hinterlands which shift in shape as well as being largely tacit, unclear, and impure.[67]

Donna Haraway's understanding of knowledge as situated hints at a similar appreciation of the entanglement of social construction and scientific objectivity. For Haraway, there is a deep appreciation of the need for a radical constructionism where all forms of knowledge claims—including science—are socially constructed and specific to the places and times in which they develop. Yet she also sees the need for something more: "a no-nonsense commitment to faithful accounts of a 'real' world," or at least "one that can be partially shared and that is friendly to earthwide projects of finite freedom, adequate material abundance, modest meaning in suffering, and limited happiness."[68] Such real but only partially shared worlds are the object of study for anthropologist Anna Tsing, who studies global changes through concepts of awkward engagement between traveling realities.[69] In this mode of thinking, I approach hygiene as a traveling cultural practice that is deeply embodied and deeply enculturated, as illustrated by the empirical work in this book. Still, there is something in it to be shared: an account of health, wellbeing, and guarding life based on a partially shared human body and a partially shared planet, and the objects, structures, and institutions assembled around it. Hygienes, like diseases, can travel, but they may not travel in the ways we are trained to expect through tidy accounts of public health campaigns.

Understanding hygiene as a situated assemblage is helpful because we are then set free from understanding hygiene as a set of universal best practices (such as handwashing or diaper use). This allows us to move toward understanding the contextual and situated development of hygiene practices while attending to flows of power. The ways in which the configurations of hygiene assemblages unevenly ebb and flow and reorganize over time, both intentionally and unintentionally, also provide insight into the processes and possibilities of hygiene and sanitation as assembled in other modernities, ontologies, and epistemologies. Becoming aware of the current diversity of hygienes works to multiply possible (hygiene) futures in that within this diversity of practices and assemblages may lie other possible hygiene futures already partially enacted. Paying attention to these diverse, situated hygiene assemblages provides us with the means to examine our own hygiene assemblages, wherever we might be, particularly those that may be environmentally harmful even as they protect against harmful bacteria or viruses.

In what follows, we take a deeper dive into hygiene assemblages in China. China is an ideal place to study diverse hygienes, with its long history of written health texts and a well-documented history of governance. For readers from and in the Western world, this is important because it helps us see an alternative hygiene assemblage in a full, real, and positive way. It helps us witness an existing functioning hygiene reality that is different from (yet overlaps with) those assumed, imagined, and experienced by United Nations Development Programme project managers as they track indicators. For readers from elsewhere in the world, particularly the majority world, it provides a point of entry for examining forms of place-based hygiene that already exist elsewhere and everywhere. For readers from China, I hope it provides an opportunity to rethink and revalue what is sometimes thought of as *luhou,* backward, and instead carefully consider how good health might be guarded in the context of rapid social change.

In the Courtyard of Venerable Grannies

2007. Xining, China. The communal courtyard of my *xiaoqu,* or block of apartments, is always busy. There are six long buildings, three on each side of a central walkway, with courtyards between them, with about three hundred apartments altogether. Unlike the urban anonymity of the apartment blocks I inhabited in Australia, our *xiaoqu* in Xining has the feel of a village or an extended family. Older residents frequent the communal areas, playing mah-jongg and Chinese chess, drying chilies on large tarpaulins, and making pickled cabbage in giant clay jars. They would garden, exercise gently, rock babies, or knit while watching older children play. Small children often toddle around, invariably dressed in split-crotch pants, often in several padded and colorful layers. This style of dress keeps the legs of babies and toddlers warm while making it easy to hold them out to urinate, or for them to squat and urinate independently without wetting their pants.

My daughter is also a toddler, so I take her down to wander around the courtyard, letting her curiosity lead our meanderings. We might see a grandmother encouraging her small charge to squat and urinate on a concrete area of the courtyard, where it may be clearly seen and avoided by others. I am interested because a parent caught short in Australia or New Zealand, where I had lived most of my life, would have encouraged a child to do so on the grass.

Elsewhere, a few grandparents perch on wooden benches and small stools with their grandchildren held calmly in position, chatting to their neighbors while waiting for the child to respond to this positional cue to urinate. Around the *xiaoqu,* this action of holding out a baby is frequent, almost instinctive: a grasp under the knees mimicking the squat position used for toileting from birth to old age. Eventually a baby urinates, responding to the cue of a low whistle from a grandparent. The small puddle quickly dries in the cool, arid climate of the Qinghai–Tibet Plateau.

It is here that I begin my study of infant toileting practices in Xining. My *xiaoqu* is called Yellow South City, after a regional town some hours from Xining. This *xiaoqu* was built by Yellow South City's local government. In a way, a village has been transported here; most of the inhabitants hail from Yellow South City itself. The apartments were first made available for purchase to local government employees and retirees. In March 2007, I am renting one of these apartments while living here with my family as I begin with a total-immersion Mandarin class at nearby Qinghai Minority Nationality University. As winter melts into spring, we fall into a routine. Every day, when I return from class, I bring my daughter downstairs to the courtyard to play with the other toddlers. She grasps my hands and uses them to help her walk around and explore the large, pedestrian-friendly area. I answer interested questions from the local *nainai* (grannies), who offer me advice in every area of child-rearing. Our conversations follow a particular pattern:

GRANNY: And how old is this little treasure?
KELLY: Eight months, more or less.
GRANNY: Do you care for her yourself?
KELLY: Yes, with my husband.
GRANNY: Is he a businessman?
KELLY: No, we are students. I am doing my doctorate in Australia. I've come here to do fieldwork and study Mandarin at Qinghai Minorities' University. My husband took some time off to come help me.
GRANNY: Hmm. Where is *popo* [mother-in-law]?
KELLY: Back in New Zealand.
GRANNY: Why didn't you leave baby with her?

As far as the grannies of Yellow South City *xiaoqu* are concerned, child care is something that comes with retirement. Indeed, some express the opinion that my mother-in-law should really be retiring to take up this role. The grannies in my *xiaoqu* often interact with me, along with other mothers my age, advising (and scolding) me in all matters relating to child care as a matter of course. This includes the practice of baniao, literally "holding out to urinate." I do have some experience with this, as I had started holding out my own daughter from very early on. But until my arrival in Xining, I certainly lacked the cultural, social, or spatial support enabled by living permanently in a baniao community of practice.

The grannies provide tips on baniao, answer my questions, and monitor my daughter's clothing and food. Sometimes other people hold out my daughter when they thought she needed to go. As we laughingly stumble through communication with a mixture of speech and sign language—they with their heavily accented Qinghai Mandarin, I with my limited but growing toileting vocabulary—I get the sense that vocal communication is not emphasized for these grannies and their babies. They shake their heads in puzzlement at my attempts to explain the signs of toilet readiness taught to mothers in Australia who plan to toilet train their toddlers conventionally (one of which is being able to say the necessary words). Here, toileting is an issue separate from speech development; babies bodily communicate their toileting needs from birth anyway. It is our job, these grannies insist, to care for children's hygiene; they must pick up on children's signals and help them to an appropriate place, whether or not they can speak.

Later that month, while visiting a neighbor, I witness a grandfather sitting on the edge of a toilet seat, holding out his five-month-old grandson over the tiled floor. He laughs when I shake my head, then balance awkwardly as I try to cue my daughter toward the toilet. He points at the mop on the floor, showing me how it used for mopping up baby urine. I suddenly understand the legion of rag mops projecting out of bathroom windows, washed and now drying outdoors. I later find that cueing infants to urinate on the floor is fairly common, even in living areas, if a basin or potty is not close at hand. After my initial shock, I understand that mopping the floor is preferable to handwashing the wet garments that would ensue if baby was not quickly attended to.

Living in a baniao culture and space alongside other parents and grandparents revolutionized our own toileting practice with our infant. We enthusiastically bought a few versions of the standard toddler outfit: sets of cotton split-crotch thermal underwear, woolen or synthetic jerseys, split-crotch dungarees, and padded jacket-and-pants sets, topped with polar fleece pinnies that caught most of the daily mess of toddler living. Our baby's cute bare bottom was regularly seen flashing around the place, and we became known in the foreign community as a bit out there. But the clothing made sense in the dry, cold climate of Xining—removing a toddler's (several layers of) pants every time they need to urinate is both time-consuming and tan-trum inducing—and the split crotch made holding out the baby an effortless action.

We also began to understand the role of place in our baniao practice. Until moving here, we had not realized how inhibited we felt by Australian environment and society, with our practice mostly kept to private spaces. Although we never managed to feel comfortable cueing our children to urinate on the floor, we did eventually construct a hybrid practice of baniao that fit with our living space and habits.

2 Holding Out

Chinese people are not accustomed to using nappies, because those things—for children—cannot be endured. It seems their quality is not good.

    —Dong Mei Li, 2009

You are forever trying to keep the child dry and clean. Why? Because this skin is so sensitive. Ai, [nappies are] bad for the child's skin!

    —Lao Yang, 2009

In many places in the world, nappies are not used as the primary means of infant toilet hygiene. Digo children in the Congo, for example, are dry through the night as early as four months of age.[1] This is in contrast to North America, where children can be as old as four years of age before remaining reliably dry through the night—a state of affairs attributed by Barbara Rogoff to a cultural emphasis on children's verbal rather than non-verbal communication of toileting needs.[2] In northwest China, it is possible for babies to also be dry through the night as early as four months, although this is not expected. People clothe their young babies and older toddlers in split-crotch pants, holding them out over an appropriate spot to urinate as needed, both night and day. This practice has no specific name, but the action is referred to colloquially in Mandarin Chinese as baniao, "to hold out to urinate."[3] I use the term *baniao* to refer to the practice as practiced in China at the time of this research. Elsewhere, people have called it assisted infant toileting, elimination communication, or natural infant hygiene.[4]

In my research, I found that many people begin holding out their babies from birth, and indeed many reported that this was one of the easiest times to predict and assist eliminations, because babies are mainly held in arms. More mobile babies can also be assisted to eliminate in appropriate places, and finally toddlers start to become more independent and vocal about their elimination needs. In this method, hygiene is kept not by containing babies' eliminations against their bodies, preventing cross-contamination with other people, but by separating spaces for different embodied behaviors and uses. For example, the way one interacts with the ground and the floor in Xining is quite different from the norms in New Zealand, where I currently live. The use of separate spaces will be detailed in this chapter as I follow the practice of baniao from birth to toilet independence.

Many of the caregivers who managed the practice of baniao were grandmothers. Some of them had retired as early as forty-five to care for grandchildren, and the majority were in their fifties. As a young mother in my late twenties at the time, forty-five still seemed a lifetime away—but now, as I write on the other side of forty, I am closer in age to those grandmothers. On the one hand, it is astounding to me now that retirement would happen at this age. On the other hand, while I am coming to the end of my intensive child care years at forty-two and am finally getting my book written, for many, retirement is their first time performing daytime care work. This is because when their own children were small, their mother-in-law took responsibility for child care while they, as young mothers, went to work. For many families, this included actually having grandchildren live with their grandparents while parents worked elsewhere in the province or further afield. One family I met had twins, with one twin living at each of the grandparents' houses, and their mother would cycle first to one house and then the other to breastfeed them before going to work as a doctor. Our neighbors had two toddlers, cousins, the children of their two sons, working in the next province over as migrant workers. Migrant workers often do not have access to appropriate housing for children; they live in dormitories or even camp at the construction sites where they work. Grandparents thus take on a large load of unsupported child care in situations where parents must go out of their hometowns to work.

I talked to both grandparents and parents, almost all of whom were women. As I listen again to these recordings, I cringe at my stumbling Mandarin and feel grateful for the generous responses I received. I try to capture some of this dynamic in my interludes and in my description of what follows. My daughter is now seventeen, and many things have changed in Xining since we were last there in 2012. For one, the spatialities of hygiene, like everywhere and everything else, have been deeply affected by the Covid-19 pandemic. For another, the use of disposable nappies for infants has increased since my fieldwork—but not as much as was expected by market analysts, given increasing urbanization. Outside of China, interest in the details of baniao remains high in parenting circles, particularly among young parents concerned with the environmental effects of having a child and those whose own parents are unable to travel to assist them with a new baby as a result of pandemic constraints.

How do you keep hygiene without using nappies? In what follows, I detail answers to this question in the context of western China. I try to keep to a rich description of these practices, avoiding any unnecessary analysis to provide a sense of how it all works. I hope you can see the various strands of the hygiene assemblage that cluster around and enable the practice I describe.

NEWBORNS AND BABES IN ARMS

If you were to walk around the maternity ward of the Red Cross Hospital in downtown Xining, you might notice that the exposed piping of the central heating system is hung with oblong cotton rags of varying colors and prints. These are the *niaobu,* urine cloths, of the newborn babies you might glimpse being rocked gently by grandmothers, aunties, or fathers in adjacent rooms as the mother lies in bed, recovering from birth. The newborn baby is not generally held out to urinate but is dressed lovingly in new cotton garments with a well-worn and -washed *niaobu* of faded cotton tucked between the legs and cutesy-print, tie-up, open-crotch pants.[5]

These tie-up garments minimize the distress of dressing a newborn baby; they can be gently dressed by laying the baby on top of the opened clothing and tying it on. The soft, 100 percent cotton *niaobu* are cut from old sheets and pillowcases and are prewashed or scalded in boiling water to soften and sterilize them.[6] The *niaobu* are oblong, tea towel–size rags that are folded into a pad fifteen to twenty centimeters wide. These are tucked into the front and back of the split-crotch pants and are sometimes secured with a small band of elastic (Figure 2). The baby is then dressed in more layers of cotton, often padded or quilted cotton split-crotch suits, then wrapped in a large, cotton-filled hooded sleeping bag or quilt. Often a mink-style polyester blanket is added to this already large bundle, which is wrapped over the other layers and sometimes covers the baby's face while outdoors. Keeping newborn babies warm is a concern all over the world,

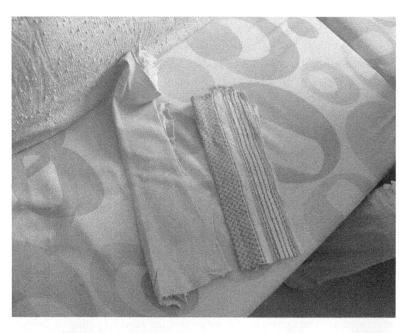
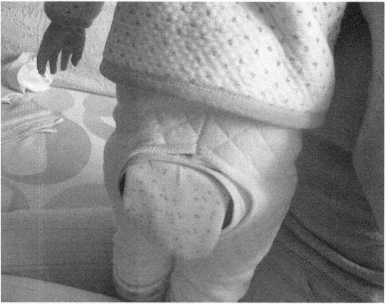

FIGURE 2. *Niaobu*. Soft cloths are tucked in the waistband of a baby's split-crotch pants. Photograph by author, 2009.

and local beliefs are strongly in favor of minimizing the baby's exposure to wind or drafts and keeping them as warm as possible with natural, soft layers of cotton.

It can be difficult underneath all these layers to change the *niaobu,* which may also leak and wet the other clothing if not changed immediately after the baby has urinated. It seems to me that it would be much more convenient, therefore, to use disposable nappies in the early days.[7] Yet from the large number of *niaobu* hanging around the hospital ward, the inconvenience does not seem to deter contemporary mothers and their attendants, who must watch the baby's body language closely to ascertain when the cloth needs to be changed. This is actually the first stage of the infant toileting process: learning the baby's idiosyncratic elimination signs and responding to them quickly and consistently in order to reinforce them.

Caregivers will respond to signs of discomfort with other actions before trying to feed the baby. If the baby is squirming, crying out, or unsettled, its carers will often first try changing the scenery, rhythmically moving (to induce sleep), or checking the *niaobu.* Sometimes responding in this way resettles the baby, who goes back to sleep without feeding, thus reinforcing communication around interactions involving sleeping and elimination.[8] If the *niaobu* is wet, the older woman accompanying the mother in her early days is usually the one to change it to a dry one, then immediately handwash the wet *niaobu* and anything else that got wet in the process. These are then hung to dry on the central heating system, or, after returning home, in the courtyard or in the *yangtai* (literally "sun platform"—a glass-enclosed balcony considered essential to newer Xining apartments, and a popular spot for wet laundry, the convalescing, the elderly, and babies).

Some families now use disposable nappies during this early period. Zhuo Ma, a Tibetan mother of a seven-month-old, says she used disposable nappies for the first two months, with the first pack having been given to her in the hospital:

> In the hospital, he only wore disposable nappies. Around the time of two months, I was in my hometown and then I didn't use disposable nappies, because disposable nappies are plastic and using them all the time is not good. Could have been around. . . . We were here [in Xining] for one month, then returned home. . . . You could say from the second month, I just let him pee independently [of a nappy]. Until this day he wears split-crotch pants

in the home, and from the time of the second month we just put a cotton *niaobu* on him [while out].

In this case, Zhuo Ma had five months off work, the first of which was spent convalescing in Xining directly after birth and the second of which was in her hometown, a village about three hours' drive from Xining. Once in her hometown, they switched from disposable nappies to *niaobu*. After another month of recovery, she and her mother started holding out the baby—or as she puts it, they "let him pee by himself." This marks the beginning of the next stage of infant hygiene management.

HOLDING OUT

Families begin holding out babies to urinate at about the first month. This time also coincides with a certain measure of infant head control, making the whole process much easier. From this time, the baby can easily be held by gripping under the thighs with both hands (the action suggested by *ba-* in *baniao*), with the baby held in an upright position with back and head resting against the carer's stomach or forearms. The baby is suspended above the ground or over a receptacle in a comfortable and secure way, and the position can be maintained easily with little pressure on the carer's back or arms (Figure 3). The relaxed position is essential in assisting the babies themselves to relax and thus release a stream of urine. In the early days, merely holding a baby in this position is enough to trigger urination or defecation, and the family uses this opportunity to set up an aural cue: a low, soft whistle. Soon afterward, when the baby develops more control over the sphincter, hearing this whistle will stimulate the relaxation of that muscle and signal to the baby that now is an appropriate time to eliminate.

Babies develop different signs for impending elimination, which may change throughout the year or more of holding out. Deng Yi's seven-month-old would make a noise like "unh" when needing to pee or poo. Others, like Dong Mei Li's seven-month-old, made no clear signs, and he "always wet his pants." Guo Lihao's one-year-old would toss and turn in bed when she needed to urinate, and her mother would hold her over a basin beside the bed. One nineteen-year-old ethnically Hui[9] university student who lived above his grandparents' noodle shop during the holidays told me how his younger cousin (around twelve months old) would squirm on the couch and grunt in a specific way before urinating. He would then have time to lift the baby off the couch and hold him out appropriately.

Alongside signs, most families used a degree of timing in predicting when to hold out their babies. Ma Xiao Long estimated that when he was watching television with his little cousin, he tried to hold him out at least once every hour. Zhuo Ma likewise indicated that her father (who is the primary carer for her son during the day) holds out her seven-month-old every two hours. Guo Lihao told me that if her one-year-old had recently been breastfed or had drunk some water, she held her out every ten minutes. Other mothers and caregivers used timing between thirty minutes and two hours, with variations depending on the last feed, the amount of water drunk, and the type of weather.

In addition to set time periods, there were certain times of day when babies were always held out. Most common were first thing in the morning and after any naps; other times included after drinking, before going out somewhere, and if the baby had not urinated in a while. If the babies did not want to urinate, they would look uncomfortable or arch their backs,

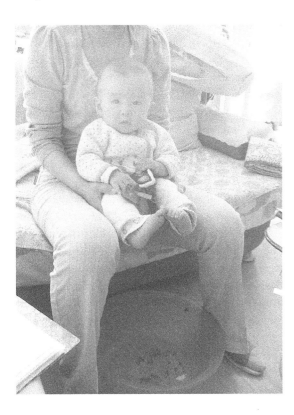

FIGURE 3. Holding a baby over a potty basin. Photograph by author, 2009.

clearly showing refusal. Some families respected refusals even though they were pretty sure the baby needed to eliminate, and merely tried again later. For some families, their stronger-willed children went through long periods of back arching and wet pants. Others (often grandparents) thought that in certain circumstances, babies should be grasped firmly and kept in position until they responded. This strategy was most often pursued when outside or on the balcony, where babies could look around and sit peaceably until something happened.

During the night, around half of the babies whose mothers or grandmothers I interviewed wore disposable nappies, which allowed parents to be less responsive—and, they hoped, get more sleep. Most of the babies urinated two to three times during the night, and even the mothers I interviewed with babies in disposable nappies still mentioned waking up and knowing when the baby was urinating. All the babies slept alongside someone, normally their mother or both parents but sometimes with grandparents. Babies not in disposable nappies were placed on a thick but firm cotton-stuffed sleeping pad in case of accidents. Guo Lihao's baby slept on such a pad but mostly stopped urinating at night at around two or three months of age (despite one or two night feeds). At the time of the interview, her baby was one year old and frequently feeding at night (being more distracted during the day), yet she still rarely had to get up to baniao.

A niaobu was also used when disposable nappies were not, although this did not prevent urine from leaking onto the pad or bed. Zhuo Ma, the Tibetan mother of a seven-month-old, thought this was easier in rural Qinghai homes where families slept on heated brick platforms known as kang. Here, a damp sleeping pad would be turned over and would quickly dry during the night. In urban situations, the quilt would be changed, or a layer of towels or rags would be used on top of the quilt and these changed instead, leaving the quilt only slightly damp. The quilts would then be washed in the morning and hung to dry in preparation for the next night. These were some of the most ubiquitous items of laundry in my xiaoqu, probably meaning that nighttime accidents were not uncommon. And if this quilt permitted leakage onto the mattress? According to Han migrant mothers Lao Yang and Xiao Shi, the mother would sleep on the wet patch and move the baby onto the drier side of the bed.

Almost all the babies were expected to defecate first thing in the morning. This was encouraged by giving babies a large drink of warm milk or a long breastfeed. Then someone in the family would generally sit and hold the baby out until defecation occurred. Having the bowel movement over for the day created a degree of freedom for the rest of the day, as the carers could be pretty sure that they would only be dealing with relatively sterile urine accidents. Some, such as Yang Shanshan, a university lecturer and mother of a seven-month-old, thought that holding out the child too long to defecate might "pressure" the child too much and cause some "psychological problems," so she held the baby out for a maximum of three minutes, then tried again at regular intervals. Her baby generally had a daily bowel movement later in the day.

Babies were generally held out over a large, wide plastic basin used specifically for the purpose of catching urine; other, similar basins were assigned to foot washing, clothes washing, vegetable or dishes washing, and hand, face, or hair washing (for families without bathrooms). This basin was kept in a prominent position in the main living area. In some families, such as Deng Yi's and Lao Yang's, the baby was held out over the tiled floor in the living room. This was considered more convenient than emptying and washing a basin (which may end up being left unemptied, causing a smell). The puddle could be mopped up immediately. The mop only had to be cleaned every day or so, and was otherwise poked out the bathroom window to air.

Other families held the baby out over the bathroom floor, sitting on a Western-style toilet with the seat down and holding the baby out over the tiled, drained bathroom floor. The basic rule of thumb appeared to be as follows: hold out the baby somewhere light, easy to clean, and with interesting things to look at, in a position equally comfortable for baby and adult. This often excluded holding babies out over toilets or sinks, which in Xining are often in windowless, cramped rooms that do not assist with baby relaxation or adult comfort.

In some basic rental homes, there is no toilet. In Guo Lihao's fruit shop's back bedroom, Xiao Shi's vegetable shop's back storage room, Ma Xiao's rented room in a shared courtyard, and Zhang Li's wine shop with its loft bed, the babies did their daily bowel movement on several layers of newspaper on the floor, which was then wrapped up and disposed of in the daily commercial district rubbish collection. In fact, even people with bathrooms sometimes used this method, as it allowed the adult to sit comfortably while the baby defecated, and it also minimized (or even eliminated) the contact required with feces. The paper could be shaken into the toilet and then thrown away, rather than having to scrub out a potty or basin.

Yang Shanshan, whose baby was the only one not made to defecate every morning, described a time when she and her husband realized while out that their baby needed to poo. They quickly bought a newspaper, placed it on the side of the street, and held the baby over that. She found the experience "very embarrassing." This is an interesting case to note, as many Western observers assume that the holding out of babies over gutters goes for both kinds of eliminations, but clearly this is not the case.

Once babies are old enough to hold out, even when they are wearing a *niaobu* or a disposable nappy, they are rarely just left to urinate in it (during the day at least), and they are never left to defecate in it. If a baby was thought to have begun defecating, the nappy or *niaobu* would be removed, and the baby would be held out for the remainder. Some domestic brands of disposable nappies were in fact designed along lines similar to *niaobu*— long sanitary pad–type nappies with sticky areas at either end for tucking into split-crotch pants, allowing carers to hold out their babies regularly but providing some backup. Zhang Li, a Han migrant from an eastern province, lived and worked with her husband in a small alcohol-and-cigarette store while caring for her eight-month-old baby. Sometimes she found it convenient to use these nappy pads while looking after her baby in the shop. She said her baby

> uses disposable nappies, but they are just used on a temporary basis. Sometimes when I don't know [if he needs to go], or he has diarrhea. You don't want to use it, but also don't want him to poo his pants, [so then we] use one of these [nappy pads] and every now and then hold him out.

Sometimes she would get to the end of the day and throw the nappy out without its having been wet or dirtied, so her holding out had been successful despite her baby's loose bowels.

ON THE MOVE

While younger babies normally had *niaobu* (or a disposable nappy pad) tucked into their pants to absorb any accidents, these were used less often as babies got older. *Niaobu* are not overly absorbent, so in no way do they equal a nappy in terms of protecting people and places from elimination. Once babies began moving around a lot more, the *niaobu* also did not offer much benefit, and their use were discontinued as soon as babies could walk with assistance. Although Guo Lihao did not use disposable nappies at night with any of her three children, she did use them with her youngest during the earlier months while visiting friends; she thought that when the baby's pants were wet (from a leaking *niaobu*), it would feel uncomfortable. But at home,

> you don't need to use nappies. If clothes get wet, you can change them immediately—it is very convenient. Because of that, normally people don't use nappies [at home]. . . . When she is a little over a year old, or can walk and squat, I don't use any nappies, because when she can squat down, she can pee or poo by herself then.

Older babies generally wore several layers of split-crotch pants, with cotton long underwear closest to the skin, topped by hard-wearing split-crotch pants or dungarees made from materials such as denim or corduroy (Figure 4). Sometimes the child would also have hand-knitted woolen or acrylic pants between these layers. In the winter, pants would often be immediately changed if they got slightly wet during the baniao process,

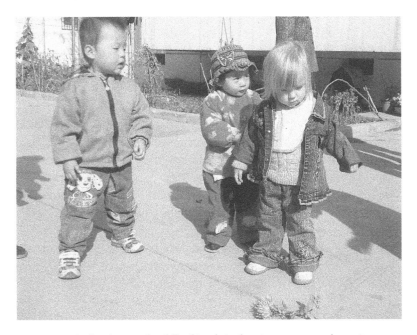

FIGURE 4. My daughter and toddler friends in the *xiaoqu* courtyard wearing typical toddler clothing. Photograph by author, 2007.

but during the summer, they could be left to dry if they were not directly touching the baby's skin.

Because few people had washing machines, baniao practice and the wider hygiene care assemblage were informed by the necessity of handwashing all clothing. Most interviewees did some washing every evening, although older children and adults each handwashed their own undergarments and socks every night. Mothers or grandmothers tended to be responsible for washing out the baby's clothes. Larger soiled items such as jackets, jeans, quilts, and knitwear were often washed by the professional laundries common on every street.

Smocks were thus an extremely important element of children's clothing in Xining, and as a result, they were often very dirty—their job being to protect the cleaner, more difficult-to-wash clothes worn underneath. Likewise, hard-wearing fabrics such as denim, corduroy, and nylon were preferred as outer layers, as these could be brushed down rather than needing to be washed like the stretch knits popular for babies in Western countries. Caregivers also used spatial strategies to prevent their children from getting dirty, such as preventing them from sitting on the ground or touching dirty items. In addition to all this, children had their faces and hands wiped frequently to prevent the transfer of dirt into other spaces.

In the city, girls often stopped wearing split-crotch pants between twelve and eighteen months of age, whereas boys were more likely to wear them until two or even three years old. In the countryside, all children wore split-crotch pants until much later, as they spent more time outdoors, out of arm's reach of their carers. Two mothers of teenage children I interviewed had generally left their children in split-crotch pants until three and four years old, respectively, implying that there have been some changes over time. The gendered differences in the length of the use of split-crotch pants appeared to be related to several things. Some Hui Muslim families thought that girls should be covered while in public starting at around this age; some families from varying nationalities and religious traditions thought that it was cleaner for girls to wear ordinary pants once they were playing independently (referring to the differences in genitalia). Many agreed that girls were less likely to wet themselves than boys at this age.

The downside of switching to ordinary pants is that the children were still unable to remove their own pants until around age two, so they would remain dependent on their parents to help them go to the toilet. This is increasingly less of a concern as people have fewer children and the adult-to-child ratio remains high.[10] In all cases, there was considerable flexibility and variance regarding the use of split-crotch pants—for example, a baby might wear split-crotch pants at home and ordinary pants while out, or split-crotch pants when one family member was caring for them but not another.

Almost all families expected significant control over the bladder and bowels by the age of one, although there was a lot of variance regarding how much control was expected. Many families expected children to occasionally urinate on the floor until they were walking confidently and could easily make it to the bathroom and squat independently over the in-ground toilet or a potty—which appeared to be around two years old. In my upstairs neighbors' apartment, which had an unfinished concrete floor, I witnessed a two-year-old pull down her pants and urinate on the lounge-room floor. She was briefly and gently scolded and told to go the bathroom to urinate, and the puddle was promptly mopped up.

Despite the apparent independence of children from an early age, most families took responsibility for managing children's eliminations until they were at least two, and often older. One Hui mother still woke her six-year-old and told her to go toilet if she was tossing and turning in their shared bed, to prevent bed-wetting. Wang Ping, a Han mother of a teenage girl, commented on the whole process in retrospect:

> Well, after a longer time, you can call out "quick, go and pee." She would understand and then pee. Well, she did OK. If she got her clothes wet, then you just changed them. After all, she was just a child. It was natural for her to wet her clothes. Just wash the clothes and change her into some new ones. Wash her wet trousers and dry them in the sun. . . . It was not troublesome, no trouble at all. This is just what you have to do. No trouble.

In summary, the journey from birth to toileting independence is marked by a number of stages: the first ritual month of lying-in, where babies' elimination habits and timings are observed; the second period of holding out, where babies are responded to and themselves respond to different cues, signs, and signals; and the final period of walking and squatting, where increasing toilet independence is expected and achieved. At each stage, caregivers strive to keep babies' bodies clean and dry, with a minimum of fuss and laundry. Although there were differences between families of different income levels, living spaces, and education, the fact remains that no families used disposable nappies exclusively, and no families regularly used more than one a day after the first few weeks. The journey to toileting independence is not an individual one, or even a household one. The description I have given so far has highlighted shared expectations around the use of public and private spaces, the material infrastructures and objects that are part of the care and hygiene assemblages, and the variety of actors involved in enabling a process of toileting individuation.

There are two elements of the assemblage that I have not yet highlighted in great detail. One is the understanding that disposable nappies are more than a singular hygiene object. They are also an object around which finance, corporate ambition, environmental concerns, and infant development come together in an overlapping global hygiene commodity assemblage. The second element is more entangled and rich in history and comprises the set of traditions drawing on understandings of *weisheng*, hygiene, and guarding life from antiquity to today—an assemblage of health-keeping practices that gathers in particular around the infant body and the body of the birthing and breastfeeding mother. I turn to each of these in the following sections to help flesh out what the full assemblage consists of, as well as to answer the question of why the intensive marketing promotion efforts of disposable nappy companies has not shifted the assemblage quite as much as their shareholders may have envisioned.

DISPOSABLE NAPPIES

The most heavily marketed disposable nappy product in China is the Procter & Gamble brand Pampers. The very name hints that Pampers are meant to pamper the baby's skin with their soft and luxurious product. Yet in Xining, this is far from accepted truth.[11]

Procter & Gamble has come under fire in recent years for their tissue products, which continue to be partially sourced from virgin forests. Shareholders voted for a change in policy, but there has been little shift in sourcing these particular products. The company has generally approached environmentalists and environmental policymaking positively, as has been the case with other activist groups that have engaged with them. For example, the company has been proactive in making sure it is not advertising alongside objectionable content, like that created by white supremacists. It maps out different environmental projects on its websites, showing where water is saved or solar power is used in factories. But the company is simultaneously committed to growing its brand and the use of its products at a global scale, and this includes disposable nappies. It has conducted multimillion-dollar campaigns seeking to increase the use of disposable nappies in China and India. It has conducted research on nappy use and has put a considerable amount of resources into convincing people in China that their children will be smarter if they use their nappy products.[12]

In some circles, disposable nappy marketing is seen as comparable to the infant formula marketing of the 1970s. In 2005, Nestlé was named the United Kingdom's most boycotted company as well as the world's most irresponsible company.[13] In Nestlé's case, people have still not forgiven them for their unethical formula marketing strategies in the 1970s, in which white-coated salespeople handed out samples to mothers in African hospitals. Their blatant miseducation endangered the nutrition of some of the most at-risk babies in the world, resulting in what is seen by some as "the largest uncontrolled clinical experiment in human history."[14] In response to increasing concerns over the role of infant formula in malnutrition and diarrhea-related deaths in the developing world, in 1981 the World Health Organization released the "International Code of Marketing of Breast-Milk Substitutes." This voluntary code requires signatories to cease the promotion of breast-milk substitutes to infants (although not to toddlers). Most multinational formula-producing companies are now signatories to this code, and it is widely supported as necessary in affirming the importance of breast milk for babies everywhere in the world.

Although disposable nappies are not as damaging to children's health as is the use of formula in vulnerable communities, their marketing techniques are increasingly distasteful in a world where excess waste is becoming an international and seemingly insurmountable problem. Trying to create a market for their product in a situation where there is barely enough landfill space to meet current demand is certainly problematic—not to mention the concerns surrounding the plastic involved in packaging and pull tabs, as well as the energy expended in production and shipping and the forests of trees used to make the softest nappies. In addition, a similar campaign of miseducation has been conducted, with companies funding research that finds the environmental impact of disposable nappy use to be comparable to that of cloth nappies. For example, in 1991, the Women's Environmental Network in the United Kingdom commissioned an independent review of the available research on the environmental impacts of disposable versus cloth nappies. The review found that all studies to that date had been funded by the disposable nappy industry, making their claims of comparable impact between the two nappy types dubious, to say the least.[15] The consultants then carried out additional research that found that disposable nappies use twenty times more raw materials, three times more energy, and twice as much water, and generate sixty times more waste. With reference to this, the Women's Environmental Network challenged Procter & Gamble's claim of environmental equivalency before the United Kingdom Advertising Standards Authority, which forced Procter & Gamble to withdraw their claim.[16]

If we were to take the health of the environment as seriously as the health of babies, it is entirely possible that an "international code for the marketing of disposable nappies" would also be issued. As it is, subsequent studies on the environmental impacts of disposable nappies have been dogged with controversy over the parameters of the life-cycle analysis techniques used.[17] Australian researchers from the University of Queensland were dissatisfied even with the assumptions about cloth nappy use in the Landbank Consultancy report. They conducted a detailed life-cycle analysis of their own based on Australian conditions such as low-water-usage washing machines and the prevalence of outdoor line-dried laundry. Their findings are even more strongly in favor of cloth nappies than the subsequent Environment Agency report; however, 95 percent of Australian babies are nappied in disposables.[18] It is possible that the environmental impact could be reduced even further because even this study excludes the widely used modern cloth nappies, which use significantly less cotton than traditional Australian terry flats or New Zealand flannelette squares. Indeed, a United Nations Environment Programme review of nappy life-cycle assessment research pointed out that families could control these conditions depending on their level of ecoconsciousness.[19]

However, what if using disposable nappies is not just bad for the environment but also for babies' health? A number of studies in the West have suggested possible links between disposable nappy use and a number of health issues, including the aggravation of asthma and chemical-related nappy rashes, not to mention a considerable rise in toilet training age over the last sixty years, which is thought to be linked to dysfunction of the lower urinary tract.[20] There are also more sinister baby health scandals linked to disposable nappies. In 2010, Procter & Gamble introduced their new Dry Max technology into their Pampers line, which was quickly followed by thousands of complaints from parents claiming that it caused rashes and bleeding blisters in their babies. The subsequent lawsuit was settled in June 2011 with payouts to parents including coverage of their legal fees and a commitment to updating the Pampers website with tips on treating nappy rash and funding for a training course for pediatric resident doctors on baby skin health. There are also cases of more serious chemical burns and skin reactions occurring when disposable nappies burst, which have been reported with Pampers and other brands. In one case, a family lost custody of their children for eight months until an independent consultant could prove to doubtful doctors and police that serious burns on a two-year-old were caused by chemicals in bursting nappies.[21]

Among the mothers and grandmothers I interviewed in Xining, research papers and manufacturing scandals are not necessary for them to know that disposable nappies are bad for children's health, and in particular the health of their skin. In fact, this is one of the biggest reasons for limiting nappy use and continuing the practice of baniao, in conditions of both poverty and affluence. Yet Procter & Gamble have tried to break into the Chinese market by sidestepping the health concerns and targeting two of the other big issues in parenting: sleep and child development.[22] Their multibillion-yuan campaign to change the nursery habits of millions of Chinese consumers has won them praise from marketing experts, if not environmentalists.

In a nutshell, after a failed product launch in 1998, Procter & Gamble partnered with the Beijing Children's Hospital Sleep Research Center to conduct home-visit research on more than one thousand babies in eight cities. Their findings were that babies in disposable nappies fell asleep 30 percent faster and slept on average thirty minutes longer (although it is not clear whether this comparison was with the same baby without disposables or with the average of alternatively nappied / nappy-free babies). The company lost no time in linking this extra thirty minutes' sleep to brain development—a particularly astute move in a society where academic achievement is highly valued—and began the viral Golden Sleep campaign. Parents uploaded photos of their sleeping children to a website, which were then used to create a huge photo montage in a Shanghai department store as part of the marketing campaign. The company also made sure their product felt soft and light and less plasticky, imitating the soft cotton feel that is an important characteristic of *niaobu*. The campaign seems to have done its job well: Procter & Gamble's Pampers brand has been one of the top-selling brands of disposable nappies in China. Yet even Procter & Gamble admitted that most of its customers only used one nappy a day.[23] The rise in nappy use in the last few years has been long in coming, but it has also shifted toward local designs that support baniao alongside nappy use. One thing Procter & Gamble did get right, however, was that the core concerns of caregivers in China were not absorbency and/or cheapness, as had first been assumed, but about quality and the feel of the product against the skin. The next part of the hygiene assemblage I will address is that of traditional Chinese medicine (TCM) and ideas around skin and baby health more generally.

THE IMPORTANCE OF BABIES' BOTTOMS

The baby's bottom is tai nen, "very delicate," and must be cared for attentively, at least according to Han migrant grandmother Lao Yang. As soon as the niaobu gets wet, it must be changed, she said, noting, "You are forever trying to keep the child dry and clean." As soon as the baby is able to be comfortably held out, this is the preferred option for all eliminations because it means that the baby's delicate skin does not have to come into contact with either feces or urine. While baby urine was considered relatively harmless—and in some cases even medicinal—the idea of a baby sitting in a damp nappy was objectionable, and in a soiled one, inconceivable.[24]

To avoid this dampness, Deng Yi changed her baby's nappy up to three times during the night when he was younger and still urinating frequently. Zhang Li used niaobu until around 11 o'clock at night, then used a disposable until morning, when she "threw it [down] and let the baby pee on top of it." Although it was well accepted that disposable nappies somehow "draw away" the urine from the baby's skin, every person I talked to thought that even so, dampness was present and was contained against the skin because the nappy did not breathe. Deng Yi said, in regard to disposable nappies, "Just sticking them in disposable nappies, that kind of sealing up I think is not good—too airtight!" She preferred to use niaobu despite appearing to live in circumstances that would enable her to afford disposable nappies. Her concern with nappies, then, was not so much that the baby was sitting in urine or feces for any length of time but that the very nature of nappies was to "seal up" and be "airtight," stopping the flow of air around baby's bottom. This was considered bad for the baby's skin, even if the nappy was clean.

The concern for keeping air flowing around the baby's bottom was evident in Xiao Shi's comparison of niaobu with Western-style cloth nappies. Xiao Shi was an experienced nanny or baomu and has come into contact with many Western baby-care practices during her time in Xining. She discussed the differences between Western and Chinese cloth nappies with Deng Yi and me:

XIAO SHI: Our *niaobu* are different from yours [directed at me]. Yours are thick, pretty thick. Ours are comparatively simple. Just a whole lot of squares [of cloth], a whole pile. Theirs [directed at Deng Yi, indicating me], you would notice, are really thick! Ours are pretty much like this one here [indicating Deng Yi's son], all are cotton, one layer at a time, and of the same size as disposable nappies. They are homemade, or you can also buy.

DENG YI: Ours have just one layer, very thin. It should be changed right after it is wet.

XIAO SHI: So that the babies are comfortable.

DENG YI: If it is too thick, although it won't leak, he will feel uncomfortable.

XIAO SHI: Babies' bones and flesh are all soft. Their legs might become deformed [if it is too thick].

While Deng Yi and Xiao Shi were both concerned with the thickness of Western nappies causing discomfort by stopping airflow, Xiao Shi also alludes to another older custom in some areas in China and Central Asia where babies' legs are swaddled straight to prevent deformity.[25] She did not swaddle her babies because this is not common practice anymore, but she still harbored a concern for anything that might hold babies' legs apart in a set position. In Xining, it was the custom to carry babies high, with their legs held tightly together, half-seated on the arm of the adult, rather than low and over the hip as many Westerners do. In fact, this position over the hip was probably enabled by nappies; I discovered it was uncomfortable with a nappy-free baby. The legs-apart position is a cue for babies to eliminate, so it would hardly be appropriate for carrying small babies, yet there was still an underlying concern that constraining the baby in this position with nappies might be innately damaging to the hips or legs.

Disposable nappies were thus, in some aspects, considered more appropriate than Western-style cloth nappies, at least in terms of the width between the legs, which allowed the legs to come together in the preferred position for carrying Xining babies (Figure 5).

Disposable nappies were still of concern because of their plastic content, which not only reduced airflow and contributed to their airtight quality but were also nonnatural, factory-made products carrying the potential of contamination or danger. In one interview, Zhang Li alluded to a nappy-manufacturing scandal, saying she preferred the Anerle brand over Queshi because she had read in a newspaper article that the "brand was not good." In light of recurring quality scandals in a variety of manufactured products, let alone the Pampers scandal in the United States, it is not unreasonable for caregivers to worry about the potential of disposable nappies harming babies in some way.[26] Caregivers were not thinking about the dangers of contamination in this case but rather the overall health of baby's skin and the circulation of blood and qi.

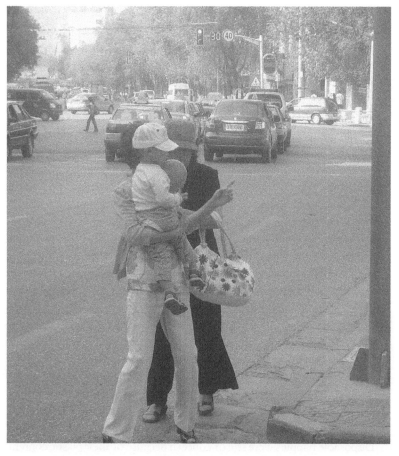

FIGURE 5. Usual position for carrying a baby in Xining. Photograph by author, 2009.

In Xining, nappy rash was considered unusual and abnormal. Including plastic as a guard against leakage was not necessarily a good thing in the eyes of many caregivers because it could lead to nappy rash. The Anerle nappy pad is preferred among many local mothers as being a sort of disposable version of the *niaobu,* allowing frequent removal and baniao opportunities as well as increased airflow due to its less constricting design. Although it still appeared to contain a plastic backing, this was less worrisome because it was not pressed against the baby's bottom.

In addition to concerns about the babies' bottoms and their delicate skin being prone to rashes, keeping the area overly damp and hot created other health and skin-related concerns. Zhuo Ma noted that it was not appropriate to use disposables while sleeping on a heated *kang* in her home village; the plastic, combined with the warm *kang,* meant that "blood cannot go smoothly in its vessels." She thought that not only was cloth more comfortable (as long as it was changed promptly) but it also protected the child's health in other ways. Here she alluded to coagulated blood, a condition recognized by both traditional Chinese and Tibetan medicines. If the blood is coagulated, or not flowing smoothly, there is a danger that this will allow the development of stagnant, damp heat, which in TCM is indicated by redness around the two yin (genitalia and anal areas). According to *A Handbook of TCM Pediatrics,* this "nappy rash" is a symptom of damp heat and not necessarily a condition in and of itself.[27] Damp heat can migrate, causing other health problems, many skin related (such as cradle cap or eczema) and some gastric related (nighttime colic and continuous abdominal pain).

On the one hand, although many would assume rural families are less likely to use disposables because of economic constraints, it is just as likely that in northern and northwest China, families with *kang* avoid disposables at night because of damp heat concerns. On the other hand, Zhuo Ma thought that using disposables in the city was more appropriate because the bed was not heated and a *niaobu* would quickly become cold when wet. In other warmer and damper areas of China, disposable nappy use was also reduced in the summer, presumably because of similar concerns about damp heat. Babies' bottoms are more than just a delicate area of skin; they are an important temperature-regulating area that must be kept clothed in natural fibers with some airflow permitted.

Because of the reasons discussed above, disposable nappies were therefore not always desirable, even if supposedly more convenient. In fact, many people I talked to thought that using split-crotch pants was actually more convenient in that it allowed this important area of skin to be cared for without the hassle of constant nappy changes. Nappy changing becomes more and more difficult as children grow and become more mobile, and this, combined with the lack of nappy-changing facilities in Xining and the comparative ease of mopping up urine from tiled floors, meant that disposable nappies were really only considered useful during the night, if then. The benefits of the baniao method of infant hygiene were considered to far outweigh its disadvantages; some considered it to have no disadvantages at all, although others thought it had the one disadvantage of being bad for the environment (meaning the cleanliness of the domestic and urban environment). This element of the hygiene assemblage includes long traditions of baby care that prioritize airflow and tender care of the baby's delicate bottom. Indeed, although the brand name Pampers is presumably meant to refer to the pampering of a baby's delicate bottom, in Xining, it is more likely to refer to pampering the inanimate home and street, the *huanjing* or (immediate) environment, because any caregiver seriously wanting to pamper a baby's bottom would be committed to the practice of baniao.

HOLDING OUT UNIVERSAL BOTTOMS?

None of the reasons for preferring baniao to disposable nappy use are limited to Xining babies' bottoms. Although occasionally Xining women excused the apparent ignorance of foreigners with regard to health practices with a shrug and the statement "our bodies are different," for the most part, people believed that the characteristics of babies' bottoms and bodies were universal. Anyone who looked closely at Western children's illnesses could probably find evidence of problems of damp heat, related both to Western clothing and nappying practices and Western diets (high in wheat, dairy, red meat, and sugar—foods that, according to TCM, stagnate in the immature digestive systems of children and babies and do not help produce quality breast milk). In the same way, people in the Western world also imagine a universal baby body. In this universalist imagination, Western commentators insist that in the case of baniao, "it is the parent being trained, not the baby" because they cannot imagine babies controlling their elimination.[28]

Most research on toilet training in the biomedical literature is based on Western practices. Because most babies in Western nations are currently kept in nappies until at least the age of two, this age becomes the normal starting point for any research into toilet training.[29] Through the exclusion of abnormal practices in toilet training research (such as infant toileting), Western biomedicine has come to assume that the sphincter muscle (which enables one to hold on when needing to urinate) is not mature until around two.[30] From here, a subtle slippage occurred between research and general practice, where the fact that the sphincter muscle in Western children is not well developed until around age two becomes entwined with the belief that the sphincter muscle *cannot* be developed until around age two.[31] Research and practice thus perform and enact a reality where babies' sphincter muscles are not developed until age two, when toilet teaching begins in most Western cultures.

Here we see there are multiple babies' bottoms, and that caregiving practices are part of a wider assemblage that enacts different sorts of hygienes and different sorts of bodies. My ethnographic research in Xining shows that babies are able to control their own elimination needs if caregivers are willing to assist them by holding out at appropriate times; baby and caregiver are not independent, and neither is infant hygiene. The assemblage of infant hygiene practices gathered around Xining babies is one that requires the participation of both caregivers and infants. The development of the sphincter muscle is an important part of this hygiene process, but its development is something that is enacted (or not enacted) rather than identical in each child around the world. In some ways, then, our very bodies are bounded by the scientific facts we have created, even as our facts are bounded by our experiences of the world. These histories and geographies are all part of the hygiene assemblages in which we find ourselves.

The case of baniao in western China—at least at the time of my fieldwork—is a good example of a traditional practice holding out against Westernization, globalization, and corporate marketing strategies for culture change. By continuing to literally hold out their children, caregivers in Xining are also holding out against the powerful globalization discourses that presume increasing homogeneity (or existing homogeneity, in the case of sphincter muscles). In fact, by holding out against these forces, caregivers in Xining and other parts of China provide a very real alternative to nappying practices in other parts of the world and model a different hygiene assemblage. It is partly through Chinese caregivers continuing to hold out that the Australian and New Zealand mothers I describe in later chapters have come to know about the potential of their own babies to be toiled in this way. In the case of baniao, however, there was a relatively solid consensus around the importance and delicacy of babies' bottoms. What happens when there are clashing enactments of the body or when rapid changes in hygiene norms occur? For many people in China, such as the nurse who is featured in the following interlude, health-keeping practices involve more than one medical tradition and more than one understanding of the body. Then chapter 3 will spend some time introducing two strands of medical tradition that form part of the hygiene assemblage in western China.

The Body Multiple

April 2009. Xining, China. In this high-altitude city of the far west of China, I finally arrange my first interview with a maternity nurse. I arrange to meet head nurse Zhang near the security gate of the hospital compound where she works. After we exchange greetings and news of our mutual acquaintances, she leads me into the dingy and dark foyer of an older building on the hospital grounds and takes me up several floors on the elevator. We come out into a well-lit hallway adorned with advertising by formula milk companies not so subtly disguised as parenting advice. I catch a glimpse of a room full of pregnant mothers, some with cannulas feeding oxygen into their noses, enduring a droning lecture from a nurse as they get their oxygen fix to support their high-altitude pregnancies. We turn into a small office with concrete floors and old wooden and iron furniture. A neat desk in the corner belongs to head nurse Zhang, who is the managing nurse of the maternity ward.

I begin by asking her to describe her job. She immediately launches into the techniques of teaching breastfeeding to new mothers. With her doll and fake nipple, Zhang demonstrates correct positioning and technique to me, repeating what she tells mothers in the prenatal classes she runs.

Although I try hard to follow her rapid Chinese, I quickly become confused with her use of medical terms and grammar, her language more complex than my usual interviewees. Eventually I grasp that she is now talking about the Sanlu milk crisis, which occurred in 2008. Hundreds of babies had been made seriously sick by contaminated formula that damaged their kidneys.

"Before that," she observes, "we did not realize how amazing breast milk is."

I am immediately interested, because for others I had interviewed, the crisis had not featured in their decisions to breastfeed. She knows of only two mothers in her ward who started out bottle-feeding in preparation for their imminent return to work (before the baby reaches the ritual first-month or hundred-day celebration).

"If it were in the past, she would possibly use milk powder to feed the baby if she has limited breast milk. Now, if it is so, she will ask, 'What can help me increase my breast milk?' . . . Rather than wondering which kind of milk powder is better, they now know that nothing is better than breast milk. If they feel like they do not have enough breast milk, commonly we encourage them to eat more, and still insist on breastfeeding. Moreover, allow more rest and keep up good nutrition. Here nutrition refers to protein. She should consume fairly nutrient-dense foods and keep her state of mind in good terms."[1]

I must look rather quizzical at this point, as Zhang breaks with her textbook narrative style and goes out on a poetic limb to try and explain the importance of a good frame of mind for breastfeeding.

With family members, um, her mood
. . . sometimes, she will be anxious.
This child,
she has become a mother to,
in one fell swoop become a mother
transforming her role.
This child—
she becomes aware of this child.
It seems perhaps she cannot take care of a child
It could become sick
—could this child become sick?
Could it have heart disease?
She is worried about things like this,
dispirited.
Or her relationship with her mother-in-law is not harmonious
that is, her mother-in-law
her husband's mother,
the relationship between them . . .
That is, because of financial difficulties
Or [differences in the ways in which]

To feed a child
—therein may lie some problems.
It can reveal a conflict.

Head nurse Zhang then reverts to her professional, textbook tone as she summarizes: "One thing is that they don't get enough rest. If we exclude this factor, then the rest of the cases are divided between mothers who need to eat more, sleep better, and keep in a good mood. Then we also encourage them to feed the baby more. If the baby is still hungry and the breast is empty, you can prescribe a little formula. The next feed time, let the baby breastfeed first and then if it is not enough, feed formula. If this is the situation, mother is going to have more breast milk. If not, we may suggest they drink [a particular] herbal tea."

Zhang's language becomes less sure, although again more poetic, as she continues:

If there is still none, we have some Chinese medicine.
We also use this . . .
Hmm, we have some kinds of traditional Chinese medicine . . .
Milk flowing
A letdown kind, this one
A letdown kind of Chinese medicine
She can drink those scales of the pangolin [in soup] or there are some Chinese
      medicinal herbs
Also can put those pig's trotters in
can put them in
Carp can go in
She can stew it up
Can drink the soup
This is a kind of diet therapy method
Another way is to directly eat that
Directly eat Chinese medicine
Hm
Then it's . . .
There are some like this.

Head nurse Zhang switches back to narrative: "But then there are some patients, but I haven't surveyed how many—there are also some patients

who don't achieve good results. One said her milk only equals five millili-
ters, each time only two or three mouthfuls. Then she has run out of breast
milk. She tried herbal teas and other ways but she still has limited milk.
Things like this do happen. In this circumstance, she still breastfed for five
or six months, each time only two mouthfuls here, two mouthfuls there,
as necessary. In this kind of circumstance, [the mother] can still persist."

I ask her if she had any experiences like this when she was breastfeeding
her own child.

"Of course," she agrees immediately, launching into a story of how, while
putting together the necessary finances to finalize the purchase of her home,
her milk supply dwindled over two or three days and she thought she had
to give her "more than one month old" baby supplementary feeds of formula. She attributes this to her anxiety at the time:

"Hm, probably this kind of situation was because at the time I was
extremely *fachou*."

"*Fachou?*" I ask.

"It means getting worried, aiya! So much money, what to do! What to
do? What to do?"

"Yes, it's stressful."

"Mm, it's stress. Because my milk was obviously less! We have also
noticed that with our patients' relationships with their loved ones, hus-
bands, mothers, mothers-in-law, uh . . ."

> if they have a sudden argument
> they have argued
> and that night she can't fall asleep
> after the argument she is so angry
> then the next day there is no milk
> the letdown is reduced.

Head nurse Zhang goes on to describe an embarrassing experience where
her letdown returned at work and breast milk stained her nurse's uniform
rather obviously. The mental image that this story triggers serves to high-
light the fact that head nurse Zhang embodies two women: the biomedicine-
trained health professional in her starched white uniform, and the Chinese
mother drawing on centuries of breastfeeding theory and practice, leaking
through at indiscreet discrete moments.

3 Shifting Assemblages

These alternative and indigenous Chinese discourses on *weisheng,* since they failed to meet with the approval of scholars of public health, never received their own specific and exclusive name.

> —Sean Hsiang-lin Lei, "Moral Community of *Weisheng"*

If space is . . . a simultaneity of stories-so-far, then places are collections of these stories, articulations within the wider power-geometries of space. Their character will be a product of these intersections within that wider setting, and of what is made of them. And, too, of the non-meetings-up, the disconnections and the relations not established, the exclusions. All this contributes to the specificity of place.

> —Doreen Massey, *For Space*

So far I have been mapping the assemblages of infant hygiene in place in Xining, gathered around the practice of baniao. In this mapping process, I have covered the basics of baniao, the kinds of daily practices involved in keeping it going in northwest China, the introduction of disposable nappies to the assemblage, and the pushback against their use on the grounds of babies' holistic health. I now expand the map of the assemblage into the hinterlands: the historical trajectories and ontologies of the body that have informed the way that baniao, and hygiene more generally, have assembled in this part of the world. "Trajectories" might seem an odd choice of word to describe elements of the messy assemblages of hygiene that I am attempting to map out in these chapters. But I have drawn on some good company here, and I assure you that I am not slipping into any teleological

notions of time and place where the outcomes of development and change
are already known. Instead, I am intentionally drawing on Doreen Massey's
thinking around space as a simultaneity of historical trajectories—a "throwntogetherness" that is a mapping of the present assemblage that also represents and recognizes time.[1] While mapping the socialities, spatialities, and
materialities of an assemblage, we must also recognize the temporalities
of each of these constructs. These temporalities and histories are not in
the past, however, in terms of linear time. Instead, they are here, in the
very elements of lives thrown together from whatever happens to be at
hand. Why is the spatiality of hygiene ordered in such a way in Xining and
not in some other way? Why is the sociality of infant care the way it is and
not another way? What are the materialities of care and hygiene and health
keeping, and how have they changed? These questions have led me to fascinating research materials compiled by scholars of hygiene and medicine.

I find myself still bound up in Western notions of linear time, which
informs the methodical way I have traced these trajectories; it certainly
reproduces some sense of linearity to the elements of the assemblage. I have
ordered my thinking around the two key trajectories of health keeping
that converged in my observations, experiences, and interviews in Xining.
The first of these is the tradition of Chinese medicine known as *zhongyi*,
which draws on thousands of years of medical practice and writing, and
has been formalized in the government-regulated system referred to by
researchers as traditional Chinese medicine (TCM), which can differ from
the way Chinese traditional medicines are practiced in other parts of East
Asia and the world. I trace some of the changes in this tradition of thinking about the body, hygiene, and health care, including the interactions
with what is known as *xiyi*, Western medicine, which has a trajectory of its
own: folk knowledge and tradition until its restructuring (alongside other
trajectories) as biomedicine.

Thus, in this chapter, I first map out two trajectories of health and
hygiene that converge in the city of Xining: traditional Chinese medicine, or *zhongyi*, and Western medicine, or *xiyi*, particularly in its colonial
form in the late nineteenth century. While these traditions have developed
along distinct pathways, with distinct ontologies, they have also interacted and influenced each other over the last two centuries. The third part
of the chapter traces these engagements in place and time—namely the
late Qing (1644–1911) and republican period (1912–49)—both times of rapid
change in China, where a biopolitics of hygiene came to be superimposed

on traditional understandings of guarding life. Here I draw on the work of Ruth Rogaski, who masterfully builds a picture of the changing meanings of the word *weisheng*—hygiene—in her history of hygienic modernity in Tianjin, a large city in northeast China that was historically a treaty port foreign concession.[2] I draw also on the historical accounts of *weisheng* thought and action in republican-era China, as described by historian Sean Hsiang-lin Lei.[3] Using Anna Tsing's conception of traveling universals,[4] I think about how ideas travel and come to be part of new assemblages in spaces markedly different from their points of origin. I draw on Liu Xin's construction of China as a site of global history, which itself draws on new materialist thinking and ethnographic insights to argue that "globalization as both a discursive and material force is historically produced, differently so in different social worlds," and the converse notion that "histories of different social worlds are globally made in and of specific places"—in this case, China.[5] For our purposes, this helps us imagine the hygiene assemblage as both uniquely specific to China and globally influenced and influential.

The fourth part of the chapter seeks to understand how these trajectories interact in the body—for our purposes, the bodies of infants and lactating mothers in Xining. The chapter finishes with some thoughts on how the act of articulating and describing trajectories that are part of the assemblage of hygiene offers new insights into how hygiene assemblages shift and change over time, and what this might mean for a postdevelopment politics of hygiene. By the time we conclude this chapter, I hope there will be a sense of growing understanding not just of the hygiene assemblages that support, enable, and maintain practices of baniao, but also of a vision of multiplicity and pluriversal interconnection that helps us think through social change, and a postdevelopment politics more generally. First, however, let us return to head nurse Zhang and her time of *fachou*, or worry.

TRAJECTORY 1: THE PATH OF GUARDING LIFE

A sudden argument, anger, lack of sleep—stress and *fachou* from buying a house. All these emotional elements of nurse Zhang's breastfeeding story are important to consider in the health-keeping and hygiene assemblages in the place of Xining. For Zhang, the idea that an argument or selling a house could affect breast milk supply and letdown to such a degree that supplementing with formula was necessary are not ideas from her biomedical training.[6] However, it is an important element of her understanding of the breastfeeding body, drawing on an older tradition of the body and health found in Chinese traditional medicine, or *zhongyi*. For *zhongyi*, health and disease are a matter of balance and imbalance between and within bodies and environments. A healthy person can stay healthy and avoid disease by carefully matching foods and activities with the seasons and by following a path of moderation, including keeping the emotions and spirit in a calm state.[7] Before the state became involved in the biopolitics of hygienic modernity, activities that promoted individual health were often referred to as *weisheng*, guarding life, or *yangsheng*, nurturing life.[8] Let us take a few paragraphs to return to these original meanings of *weisheng* and of maintaining good health in *zhongyi*, particularly as they relate to infant care and understandings of the body.

Keeping health in *zhongyi* has been described as something of an art.[9] Of all the arts, it most closely resembles a choreographed dance or a piece of music. The key movements in the dance are balancing of yin and yang via the flow of the vital life force qi, in accordance with the five phases, or *wuxing*. In this way,

> health and disease are directly associated with the balance of *Yin* and *Yang*. . . . *Yin* represents the passive and receding aspect of nature whereas *Yang* represents the active, advancing aspect of nature. It is believed that *Yin* and *Yang* exist at the emotional, physical, interpersonal/societal, and ecological levels. . . . The two forces are thought to be interdependent, and the imbalance between them results in disease.[10]

The ancient medical text *Su Wen* (Plain questions) puts it as follows: "*Yin* and *yang* in the human body must always be kept in balance. The predominance of *yin* will cause *yang* disease and the exuberance of *yang* will lead to *yin* disorder."[11] Women, being more yin in nature, are more susceptible to yin-excess diseases, especially at times of depleted (or yin) states, such as menstruation, pregnancy, and childbirth, when *yin qi* is predominant. Men are usually more *yang* in nature, and thus more prone to hot disorders. Through the internal flows of *yin qi* and *yang qi*, physical functions interchange from one state to another. The five states or phases are referred to as *wuxing* (where *wu* is "five") and are linked to the five elements of wood, fire, earth, metal, and water, which are in turn linked to the five major organs or viscera in the five basic systems of the human body:

The Liver (Wood) system, encompassing the Liver and gall bladder and consisting of the tissues, organs, and their functional activities pertaining to Wood, as well as tendons, eyes, tears, and the emotion of anger.

The Heart (Fire) system, centering on the Heart and consisting of the tissues, organs, and their functional activities pertaining to Fire, as well as the face, tongue, sweat, and the emotion of joy.

The Spleen (Earth) system, led by the Spleen and consisting of the tissues, organs and their functional activities pertaining to Earth, as well as the stomach, muscles, lips, mouth, saliva, and the emotion of contemplation. The breasts and reproductive organs are also linked to this system.

The Lung (Metal) system, centered on the Lungs and composed of tissues, organs and functional activities pertaining to metal, along with the large intestine, skin, body hair, nose, nasal mucous, and the emotion of grief.

The Kidney (Water) system, centered on the Kidney and formed by the tissues, organs and their functional activities pertaining to Water, along with the bladder, bones, hair, ears, spittle, and the emotion of fear.[12]

These systems interpromote and interrestrain one another in various ways. The theory of the five elemental systems is used to explain the relationship between humans and their environment. Inferences drawn between these organs, elements, tastes, directions, temperatures, and so on were often present in my conversations in Qinghai—with women of (Muslim) Hui, Han, and Tibetan backgrounds. Formalized TCM theory has, in more recent years, tried to lay out the logic of these inferences so that it can be taught and passed on, but for the layperson, these associations are deeply embedded in daily life—particularly in terms of diet—and are not necessarily directly associated with the more philosophical concepts of yin and yang and the theoretical notions of *wuxing*.

The dance between the above elements is one that emphasizes harmony in everyday life, paying attention to the environment and specific situations, then responding with appropriate actions. For example, during times where *yin qi* is predominant, such as menstruation, a woman should avoid cold foods that would augment the coldness and dampness present in her body and would make her blood become thick and phlegmatic, resulting in poor circulation. Cold foods are those both literally cold in temperature and those cold in nature—such as root vegetables, like turnips, that are associated with damp earth.[13] Consuming turnips during menstruation, therefore, could contribute to the weakening of the Spleen (Earth) system, which, combined with other factors, such as obsessive contemplation or anxiety and exposure to cold wind through washing one's hair, can result in the cold syndrome symptoms of abdominal pain and diarrhea. The natural predominance of one type of qi over another works alongside a combination of factors associated with various states (influenced by the actions and emotions of the woman and her association with her environment) to prevent or expose her to illness.

Returning to the concept of *weisheng*, there were several traditional elements surrounding guarding life in ancient times. Rogaski uses seven specific pieces of advice from a section on *weisheng* in the Book of Immortal Celestials. Rogaski has interpreted these in a more general way. The first of these is guarding life by knowing the right time and place, which emphasizes acting in harmony with the environment, the season, the body's cycles, and life. The idea is to seek "knowledge of the patterns of space and time," which would allow a person to "guard life by 'rippling along' on the same wave with the forces of the universe."[14] For example, this can be done by facing due east when sitting or lying down in the fourth month of the year, because "the *qi* of life is in the Earthly Branch *mao*."[15] Another core practice is guarding life through dietary practices such as eating the right foods for the season; ingesting the right substances for good health and for the treatment of disease and discomfort; eating the right amounts of food; and balancing the pathogenic and medicinal natures of different foods. Many women I interviewed in Xining spoke of mutton, which they considered not good to eat while pregnant, but very good to eat when breastfeeding or treating childhood illnesses (via breast milk).

The last few practices summarized by Rogaski include guarding life with appropriate drugs, guarding life through sexual economy, and guarding life by circulating the "vitalities." Each of these categories includes many practices, but, in brief, they include the following: guarding life through drugs includes the ingestion of medicines (especially mixed herbal medicines) that correct imbalances and either cure or support patients through the disease course; guarding life through sexual economy refers to understandings of the finite nature of *jing*, or life essence, which is lost through ejaculation; and guarding life through circulating the vitalities refers to specific movements, breathing techniques, and meditations that circulate qi. In all these areas, the discourse relates to correcting, supporting, and unblocking different flows to help an individual regain harmony and balance.[16]

Returning again to nurse Zhang and her *fachou*, we might now come closer to understanding how breast milk production works in *zhongyi*. Blood and qi flow along certain channels or meridians, two of which are particularly important for breast milk production:

> Women's breast milk comes from the transformation of *qi* and blood of the *Chong* and *Ren* [meridians]. Downward flow is menstruation and upward flow is breast milk. If, after childbirth, milk is delayed or scant, it is due to insufficient *qi* and blood. When there is no milk, it is indubitably due to deficiency of *Chong* and *Ren*.[17]

Breast milk is therefore directly related to menstruation in that the qi and blood of the *chong* and *ren* meridians are transformed either into menstrual blood or breast milk (an observation linked with the recognition that breastfeeding delays the return of menses). This is why, during the traditional confinement period and beyond, breastfeeding mothers are supported in nourishing their blood in particular; this is directly related to their breast milk. Blood-nourishing foods and practices are encouraged throughout breastfeeding, and we can see some of the practices Zhang had observed where mothers sought to guard life through appropriate ingestion of pig trotters, carp, or pangolin.

Because breast milk production is conceptually linked to the *chong* and *ren* channels, a number of other related behaviors can affect the quality and quantity of breast milk. Because the flow of qi and blood in the *chong* channel relates to the (visceral) Liver, harboring the emotion of anger (also linked to the Liver) could therefore impair its flow and cause breast milk problems. Likewise, the *ren* channel is linked to the womb and the (visceral) Lungs, and therefore to the emotion of grief and the activity of worry. It thus makes sense that these particular emotions, and any other activities or foods that affect the *chong* and *ren* channels, would also affect breast milk quality and quantity. When Zhang was unable to prevent the buildup of stress and worry, it manifested in her ability to produce milk. According to historian of childhood in China Ping-Chen Hsiung, in ancient times, ten types of bad milk were possible. These were linked to a breastfeeding person's ill health (four types of bad milk), their emotional state (a further four types), or the character and composition of their milk with reference to the season (two types of bad milk, cold and hot). Therefore, a breastfeeding mother's emotional state could cause her to produce milk that was actually considered harmful to her infant.[18]

Certainly, among the women I interviewed, emotions and ill health were factors taken into account while breastfeeding. All the women who had cesarean sections reported ill health and had difficulties with breast-feeding; they thought that their milk was "watery," "not enough," or "not good quality." Others who had difficult births also linked this to their breast milk quality and quantity. When I asked Dong Mei Li if she breastfed her son in the beginning, she assented, but later, she added, "[There was] no milk, did not have milk; after I gave birth, I was not so well." She thus links her ability to produce milk with her postpartum health—which was not good as a result of a painful delivery, blood loss (and a subsequent trans-fusion), and failing to deliver the placenta in a timely manner. The loss of blood is thus linked quite clearly with breastfeeding difficulties in Chinese traditional medicine: while blood is flowing downward, it cannot be flow-ing upward and stimulating milk production.

One of the big changes in this guarding life assemblage in contempo-rary times, however, has been the introduction of formula milk. Now, when difficulties in breastfeeding require one to notice imbalances and under-take efforts to restore such balances, there is the option of supplementing a baby's nutrition through a scientifically formulated breast milk substi-tute. We will return to this point later, but for now, the main point is that for infants and caregivers, a core trajectory in the assemblage for hygiene in Xining is the "path" or "way" of guarding life (weisheng zhidao), which comprises precepts and practices for "conquering the one hundred dis-eases."[19] These precepts and practices are built on cosmological and onto-logical traditions where the body and its vitalities must be kept in harmony with the universe, where the way of weisheng, as Rogaski summarizes it, is to "guard life against depletion caused by the inevitable injuries of living itself."[20] This tradition of medicine seeks to intervene in the bodies of indi-viduals to balance out their susceptibility to disease through highly struc-tured theoretical and practical connections between bodies, their food and nutritional inputs, and their environments. It involves highly specific clini-cal encounters of identifying and discerning patterns according to ancient relationships, then assembling therapeutic interventions in a highly custom-ized way, including posture and movement as well as medicine.[21] But it also involves ancient associations, pathways, and forms of self-treatment that many of the women I interviewed drew on as a matter of course, illustrated here with nurse Zhang's interview. The dynamic trajectory of *zhongyi* and TCM joins the assemblage of keeping health in Xining, stretching back centuries but also interacting with other contemporary elements in highly complex assemblages, including Western biomedicine, to which we now turn.

TRAJECTORY 2: WESTERN BIOMEDICINE

Also present in nurse Zhang's story of breastfeeding is her role as a trained nurse in what she referred to as *xiyi*, Western biomedicine. Here, in the parts of her story where she draws on constructions of *xiyi*, the body of a breastfeeding woman is imagined primarily as that of a mammal, naturally able to breastfeed with some persistence. The main factors in overcoming breastfeeding difficulties are persistence, nutrition, and rest, with special mention given to ingesting protein. Time at the breast is important, and people having breastfeeding difficulties need to feed the baby more rather than less. Western biomedicine is now the dominant practice of medicine worldwide; it refers to medical practices built on the scientific insights of biology and physiology. It is also known as allopathic medicine, biomedicine, conventional medicine, and orthodox medicine. I use the term *Western biomedicine* because this is closest to the term *xiyi*, which is what people used in Xining when they were speaking to me. But as Sean Hsianglin Lei and other historians document, biomedicine as a global practice actually involved significant contributions from China, including the discovery of two plague bacilli in the early 1900s.[22] China was a significant site of knowledge production in biomedical public health in the early twentieth century, not least because its treaty port cities hosted multiple foreign public health regimes within different foreign colonial territories or concessions of the same city.

When practitioners of Western biomedicine arrived in China in the mid-1800s, *xiyi* understandings of the relationships between the environment, the body, and disease were not that far from Chinese understandings, particularly in terms of disease etiology. While Chinese medicine had a number of different understandings of how different forms of contagion worked, as for epidemics, the blame was usually laid on damp earth qi emanating from the place of the epidemic.[23] As Ruth Rogaski notes in her study of Tianjin, in the 1850s and 1860s, "most British physicians, like Warm Factor physicians in China, blamed disease on miasma, or a combination of miasma and invisible fermenting agents that rose from the soil or climate of a region."[24] "Miasma" was an explanation that came about when epidemics challenged the prevailing understanding of medicine and health in Europe, where ill health was understood to be an imbalance in humors. Frank Snowden recounts how when the plague spread around Europe, an explanation was required to understand how the humors of so many individuals could become imbalanced at the same time: "The orthodox explanation was that the atmosphere in a given locality had been 'corrupted,' creating an 'epidemic constitution.' Its cause was a deadly fermentation arising from decaying organic matter either in the soil or in nearby marshes and swamps. This poisonous effusion contaminated the air and sickened large numbers of susceptible people when they inhaled the poison or absorbed it through their pores."[25]

Xiyi had some significant advances in anatomy and diagnosis; it contained many more surgical interventions than were possible with *yi,* or *zhongyi*— Chinese medicine, as it came to be known. However, as David Luesink argues, what we now think of as Western biomedicine was largely as effective as many other medicines until the discovery of antibiotics and the subsequent rapid increase in survival rates for surgical patients in World War II.[26] We tend to read Western biomedicine's curative success backward in time, Luesink notes, when it was not necessarily as superior as its practitioners believed it to be when it was first imposed in colonial encounters around the world. It was *through* these colonial encounters, along with the political and economic power that the West wielded, that biomedicine was able to advance its curative powers through population-level statistics, institutions of research and medical practice, and the imposition of biopolitical regimes that both investigated and created new knowledges and realities of the body.

In a vivid example of the Eurocentrism of early colonial medical encounters, Rogaski narrates the activities of British invaders in the northeastern city of Tianjin in 1859 (when they were repelled) and 1860 (when they were victorious).[27] At the time, Tianjin residents and the invading British forces both understood disease to arise partly from the place of its origin—earth qi for Tianjian residents and miasmas for the British invaders. Tianjin had a moat around its walls that provided drainage for the city's streets, but according to the British, it was a source of sickness because of its smell. The British filled in the moat as a public health measure—as well as to protect their sensitive noses from the smell of the illness-inducing miasma. Rogaski's historical research uncovered some interesting conversations between the British invaders and the local gentry, where cross-cultural understandings of smell were discussed in a jovial manner: the British found the smells of Chinese cities offensive, while the Chinese found British people's personal smells offensive.[28] In many ways, this encounter reveals an interesting difference in approach. For Tianjin residents, one balanced out the effects of the environment on one's health by undertaking health-keeping practices such as eating foods appropriate for the season, drinking boiled water, indulging in regular healthful movements, and so on, as previously described. In contrast, for the British, the approach was one of brute force: changing the city environment in order to change one's health.

At this point, neither medical tradition had knowledge of germs, although both understood that disease could come from the environment in some way. Yet the approaches to managing potential sources of illness in this specific interaction in Tianjin illustrated the differences in thinking between the two medical cultures. Western biomedicine remains a blunt instrument that to this day focuses on reactive diagnosis and rapid, often violent actions to correct disease. Practices of guarding health in this tradition come out of a preference for action and intervention—a kind of engineering, "fill in the moat"–type energy, which pervades medical practice despite significant critique. In one such critique, Alexander Green and colleagues wrote to a medical journal, pleading physicians to prioritize relationships and discussion around people's illness, noting that "the healing tools and instruments of science are blunt and ineffective when used blindly in ignorance of the meaning and context of a patient's illness."[29]

This confidence in intervention has certainly played a role in the medicalization of hygiene and sanitation practices throughout the world, performing a conquering mode of interaction with pathogens and place, and shifting from a focus on nuanced interactions with an environment for individual health to population-level health interventions. In their book on biomedicalization in the United States, Adele Clarke and colleagues argue that Western biomedicine has undergone two key shifts since the 1890s.[30] The first is a process of medicalization, referring to a process by which more and more areas of life are drawn into the realm of the medical, seen as issues best dealt with by medical professionals rather than moral, personal, or social issues. For example, as birth became a medicalized event and shifted into hospital spaces in many places, it became increasingly governed by medical procedures and interventions rather than family, cultural, or local traditions. For much of the twentieth century, women were medically prepped for giving birth or delivery of their babies as if for surgery:

shaved, given an enema, put in a gown in a bed, and food withheld, along with detailed notes taken of blood pressure and other measurable biometrics. Each new technology adds more steps to patient preparation and treatment: synthetic hormones to induce birth, synthetic hormones to expel the placenta, continuous cardiotocography machines, IV fluids, and more.[31] These latter developments fit within what Clarke and colleagues describe as the "second shift" in U.S. biomedical practice: biomedicalization. Biomedicalization refers to an intensification of many of the same processes, but with an increasing reliance on technoscientific interventions, mass digital biometric data collection, and a shift from diagnostics based on examinations of organs and cells to diagnostics relying on genes, molecules, and proteins. This has happened throughout much of the minority world, and increasingly the majority world.

In the case of birth, this second shift results in not only the drama of being prepped for surgery but also of increased instances of surgery actually being performed in the form of cesarean sections, as well as the previously mentioned procedures. Decisions about such things are partially a result of policy rather than a result of clinician expertise or even clinical indicators, with policies made in response to statistical probabilities, whereby treatment could even precede illness according to the findings of large-scale research interventions tailored to gathering evidence for decision-makers.[32] As a countertrend, large-scale studies became necessary to provide evidence that many of the hospital-based medical interventions and policies that had been introduced were not actually helpful, in order to reverse them.[33] In New Zealand, like many countries, birth is followed by the baby's first interactions with the state: the baby is assigned a national health index number, and then, in hospital spaces, the baby is labeled and documented, often with a tag.[34] Blood samples are taken to screen for genetic disorders. Hearing and reflexes are tested. If problems are found, medicalization of this small person's life begins immediately. Medicine must act and must intervene, and as early as possible.[35] This mode of conquering and intervening at the population level has been a characteristic of biomedicine that can be traced back to its initial colonial roots in confident Eurocentric modes of policymaking—a trajectory that collides with twenty-first-century Xining and the assemblage of hygiene and health we are mapping here.

One aspect of Western biomedicine that interacts specifically with hygiene in Xining is the medicalization of child development. As Lena

Robinson points out in her 2020 book on cross-cultural child development, development psychology is Eurocentric and as a result is dominated by studies of white children in the United States and Europe.[36] The field seeks to create universal child development pathways in order to better assess and intervene in the case of disorders or developmental delays. However, because these development pathways are built on the specific norms of one cultural group, they are less helpful for others. Earlier I mentioned researcher Barbara Rogoff, who has sought to systematically examine variance in cross-cultural child development. In her book *The Cultural Nature of Human Development,* Rogoff reviews an impressive range of ethnographic and psychological research with the aim of questioning the universality of psychological child development stages. She takes the perspective that differences in child-raising practices across cultures and places are due to the different types of adults that are the end goal of these efforts. Each cultural group attempts to socialize their young into particular behavioral and thought patterns that make them mature in their particular setting. She gives the example of young toddlers in a forest community in the Congo who are able to forage and prepare food for themselves from an early age, illustrated, rather effectively, by a photo of an eleven-month-old toddler masterfully wielding a large machete over a melon-type fruit. The children are socialized by their caregivers into survival strategies for forest living—which is neither right nor wrong, backward nor forward, just appropriate for their lifestyles. A 2023 example of this is the four Indigenous children who survived for forty days alone in the Amazon after a plane crash, drawing on forest survival skills taught to them by their grandmother.[37]

Recently, research in Tajikistan by infant development specialist Lana Karasik has shown that traditional cradling techniques that restrict infant movements do not necessarily lead to delays in motor skills in the long term; nor do they prevent secure infant–family attachment.[38] The implication is that the development milestones for child psychology, which are often imagined to be universal, are in fact socially and culturally produced and situated in place and time. In Xining, quite different expectations around child development—both psychological and physical—were expressed and normalized, such as the fact that babies rarely crawled but learned to walk after being held mainly in arms, or that babies could learn to signal their need to urinate or eliminate on cue. Yet heterodox approaches to Western biomedicine and psychology such as those demonstrated by Rogoff and Karasik are not yet reflected in standardized child development models, which continue to be based mainly on the white children of the United States and Europe. Babies' growth rates have also been standardized, but the global standards were previously based on a sample of North American babies who were primarily bottle-fed. In 2004, the World Health Organization revised their standardized scales to reflect a range of groups around the world, basing them on breastfeeding rather than bottle-feeding growth curves.[39] Thus, we can see some movement toward recognizing that standardized models should not be based only a subset of people from one particular cultural and genetic group. However, it is still part of a push for universality over multiplicity.

The trajectory of Western biomedicine that forms one of the multiple strands assembled in my fieldwork is, like Chinese traditional medicine, a complex and dynamic assemblage in and of itself that draws in knowledge in ever-widening circles in its quest for universality. What I hope I have highlighted here is, first, the tendency of Western biomedicine to assume it is superior even when its effectiveness in a particular area is still questionable; and second, the tendency of Western biomedicine to adopt an active, intervening, and conquering mode aimed at the population level. These tendencies have led to significant successes in some areas of medicine but in problematic interventions and inappropriate universalizations in others.

AWKWARD ENGAGEMENTS OF TRAJECTORIES IN PLACE

Universals, and universalizations, are not found only in Western thinking or Western biomedicine. While Chinese traditional medicine has a deep appreciation of the individual body and its relationship with place, the insight that this medical tradition brings is still proposed to be universal. Academic readers trained in the humanities and critical social sciences may have what Anna Tsing calls a "curmudgeonly suspicion" of anything presented as universal.[40] She notes that we have been taught that universals are statements that really only hold true in their cultures of origin, which is a good reminder for those of us who have been brought up in dominant cultures with the power to impose our cultural universals on others. For Tsing, however, the study of universals is important because it can help us understand how assemblages can shift and change over time through the awkward engagement of new trajectories grinding against others in productive friction.[41] Indeed, Western biomedicine and Chinese traditional medicine have not developed in mutually exclusive ways, and the friction of their engagement is important in understanding the hygiene assemblage that gathers around parents and babies in the city of Xining in the mid-2000s. The friction of two or more universals in mutual engagement can lead to changes in practice, but not always for the reasons we might think. This point is important as we examine the universals of the body and medicine engaging with friction and heat in early twentieth-century China. I examine this time because it is one of obvious awkward engagement, where universals rubbed up against each other rather than sliding past each other, as they might do in contemporary times.

In the late nineteenth and early twentieth century, some of the more violent aspects of Western medicine's hygiene and sanitation regimes were being imposed on the northeastern parts of China in treaty settlements, and later, under Japanese imperialism. But as both Sean Hsiang-lin Lei and Ruth Rogaski argue, these regimes were met with some support by Chinese reformers who had studied Western biomedicine or other aspects of Western civilization. These reformers were often seeking to answer the question of why China—that great civilization of many thousands of years—had been forced into treaties and opium trade with colonial powers of the West against its will. Here, the awkward engagement was between the universal of China's presumed civilizational superiority and the opposing universal of the Western colonizers—and their likewise presumed civilizational superiority. After the imposition of trade treaties and partial colonization, many Chinese intellectuals at the time thought of China as the "sick man of Asia";[42] they referred to China's internal conflicts and warlordism, as well as the weak Qing state, as a "sickness." Yet as Jui-sung Yang writes, this soon came to be understood as not just referring to China's government but to a universal truth regarding the Chinese people as a whole.[43] Reformers sought to reform not just the state and public health systems but also the practices and habits of the bodies of the entire population. Reformers targeted the practice of wealthy women's foot-binding, the exercise habits of the middle class, eating habits at home, spitting habits in public, washing habits in private, ventilation practices while sleeping, and the domestic sharing of beds, cups, and towels, among many other things. All these were mainly to do with governing individual bodies, not governance more generally.[44] The sickness of the geobody of the nation-state became equated with the people themselves, whom reformers believed must change their habits and strengthen themselves in order to resist colonial incursions and humiliation at the hands of foreigners.

Universals of public hygiene and the body were thus being questioned, including the knowledges of Chinese traditional medicine and the new knowledges people were being exposed to by Western-trained doctors and reformers. Knowledge surrounding modernization, public health and hygiene, and Western biomedicine was also of interest during Meiji-period Japan (1868–1912), and it was Japanese translators who first began applying the word *weisheng* to refer to these interconnected ideas. When attempting to find a Japanese name for these interconnected practices of medicine technology and policing that were being implemented in the West under the rubric of hygiene, translator Nagayo Sensei followed the common Japanese practice of finding an elegant word in classical Chinese and adapting it for contemporary use.[45] In 1870, Sensei opted for 卫生 (guarding life), comprising two characters and pronounced *eisei* in Japanese.[46] When the Japanese occupied parts of China in treaty port concessions or during the Sino-Japanese war, they instituted many of their own public health practices and infrastructure. Japanese translators referred to these measures by simply pronouncing the same term, 卫生, in Chinese: *weisheng*. However, what *weisheng* now referred to was something quite different from its classical origins. It was not the protection of health or life alone, but the "particular type of government structures that are in charge of protecting the general health of the state's citizens."[47] As Lei argues, this type of public health–protecting enterprise had never been given a name in East Asia before because it was a totally new endeavor. Some scholars argued that the word *weisheng* never really fit well with the sense of public health, as scholar of public health Chen Fangzhi (1884–1969) wrote during the republican period that the term had "passed through so many hands that it has become incomprehensible," noting:

> The Japanese people have rashly translated the word "hygiene" as *weisheng*. . . . To translate "hygiene" into the Chinese language, they should have either used *jiankang xue* ["study of health"] or *baojian xue* ["study of preserving health"] . . . because the content [of hygiene] is to guard health and not at all to guard life.[48]

Despite these concerns, for the most part, the word *weisheng* was adopted. The double meaning continued to retain traces of an alternative hygiene embedded in cosmology and personal health even as it performed its new function as a symbol of China's modernity. Ruth Rogaski sees the role of the word *weisheng* as so central to discussions of China's modernity that she translates it as "hygienic modernity." She notes of her preferred translation:

> Today . . . [*weisheng*] is variously rendered into English as "hygiene," "sanitary," "health," or "public health." Before the nineteenth century, *weisheng* was associated with a variety of regimens of diet, meditation, and self-medication that were practiced by the individual in order to guard fragile internal vitalities. With the arrival of armed imperialism, some of the most fundamental debates about how China and the Chinese could achieve a modern existence began to coalesce strongly around this word. Its meaning shifted away from Chinese cosmology and moved to encompass state power, scientific standards of progress, the cleanliness of bodies, and the fitness of races. The persistent association of *weisheng* with questions of China's place in the modern world has inspired me to translate it as "hygienic modernity."[49]

Because she focuses on the word *weisheng,* Rogaski's work reveals how important this word and the idea of hygiene have been historically, especially with regarding aspirations of (a particular kind of) modernity. Therefore, what it refers to here is neither the Western biomedical understanding of hygiene nor the traditional understanding of *weisheng,* but rather something new. In Anna Tsing's terms, the friction of two universals awkwardly engaging in place produced a change in practices, a traveling of practices.

By the early twentieth century, many wealthy reformers supported the adoption of new practices in the personal behaviors and habits of Chinese people, and these drastic changes were by no means supported by everyone. As both Lei and Rogaski confirm, when the violent suppression of plagues, cholera, and other transmissible diseases was imposed by the Chinese state as they began to follow emerging Western biomedical disease-control practices, in many cases, it was a response to the ever-present danger of further colonization and imperial takeover if the Chinese government failed to contain highly contagious diseases. One clear example is the case of the Manchurian plague of 1910. This highly contagious plague had a 100 percent fatality rate and stirred panic in northeastern China. After treatment and containment via traditional *zhongyi* methods had failed, a young Malaysian doctor, Dr. Wu Lien Teh, was put in charge of dealing with the outbreak according to Western biomedical methods and his bacteriological expertise.[50] What was at stake was not only a deadly disease but also the understanding that China's failure to contain it could lead to further colonial incursions.[51]

Dr. Wu performed autopsies and examined blood samples under the microscope, which were not practices used by Chinese traditional medicine. He was able to pinpoint the plague bacillus *Yersinia pestis* as the source of the plague at a time when germ theory was far from fully accepted. While Dr. Wu is credited with adopting an early form of the gauze mask and using it for disease prevention,[52] other containment methods were brutal: people were forcibly tested on the streets and removed from their homes, which were burned alongside all their belongings.[53] People who were taken away to sanatoriums when infectious never returned. Appropriate rites for the dead were suspended, and mass cremations were held by imperial edict at the end of the winter, to dispose of the dead quickly and efficiently before the ground thawed.[54] During this time—that of the Manchurian plague as well as other illnesses that emerged soon after—*weisheng* came to be associated with the state and enforced and violent public health measures. Although Dr. Wu is celebrated as a pioneer of public health both in China and internationally,[55] at the time, he was subject to racist encounters with British and French doctors as well as the subject of suspicious conspiracy theories from local people.[56] From the point of view of the local people, Western biomedical approaches to the plague did not work because no cure was offered.[57] Wu's work was both enabled by and caught up in the geopolitics of the time, and although the institutions and processes he established were successful in containing two outbreaks of plague, they also fed into intense resentment and resistance to the Qing government and the new ways adopted from the Western world.

Those who resisted the adoption of this emerging *xiyi* biomedical management of disease included many practitioners of Chinese traditional medicine. The Manchurian plague forced these practitioners to develop their theories of contagion further, in what Lei calls the "reciprocal interactions among Chinese medicine, Western medicine and the state."[58] Lei's careful scholarship traces how the Manchurian plague showed advocates of Western medicine how it was necessary for the state to be involved in its diffusion, and how Western medicine became part of a project of state building. This culminated in the 1929 proposal from the Nationalist Party to ban Chinese traditional medicine, an event that prompted struggling traditional practitioners to be shocked into action and adopt a similar strategy of politicization.[59] As such, Lei argues, the state became "the undisputed driving force behind the history of medicine in modern China."[60] The different trajectories of Western and Chinese medicine became intricately interwoven in the body of the nation-states of first the Republic of China (1912–49) and then the People's Republic of China (since 1949). For Sun Yat-sen, the revolutionary who was at the forefront of overthrowing the Qing dynasty in 1911, to use Chinese traditional medicine was to betray the modernity the new republic was seeking to bring into being.[61] But the connection of Chinese traditional medicine and the rural poor who relied on it later made it a core part of communist politics. As Elisabeth Hsu writes, while Communist Party chairman Mao Zedong's earlier speeches rejected Chinese traditional medicine, by the time of the Great Leap Forward (1958–61), it had been adopted alongside Western medicine in a strategy to improve health access to a population of 500 million equipped with only 15,000 doctors trained in Western biomedicine. She continues:

> The Communist insistence on combining Chinese and Western medicine is unique in the history of twentieth century medicine. . . . It drew its force from its determination to overcome earlier tensions between the old and new, the Chinese and Western, the experiential and scientific, and the processes that resulted in the standardisation of TCM were thus not only revivalist and reformist, as in other burgeoning nation-states within which the middle classes and bourgeoisie were growing, but aimed at being revolutionary. The goal was to blaze a trail of integrated medicine that attended to the wants of the masses and future generations.[62]

Here we see that the universals of Chinese traditional medicine and Western biomedicine are no longer awkward but instead harmonized and apparently integrated into state-supported TCM. Scholars who find the systems integrated often find that integration rooted in the shared goal of nation building, but it is hard for me to assess the degree to which nation building was at the heart of the interactions between the two systems, or whether nation building is at the heart of scholarly interest in the early 2000s English-language literature I have been reading, which seemed to flourish after translations appeared of Foucault's work on biopower. It seems clear that both traditions of medicine claim to explain the body and how to guard its health in ways that are assumed to be universal, and for this very reason, they played a role in the building of the nation-state of China from the ruins of warlordism, imperialism, and colonial incursions of European powers and Japan. The struggle over science, ontology, and the body was part of the struggle of revolution, modernization, and the nature of the nation-state emerging from a tradition of governance and politics that had previously followed a quite different trajectory and mandate.

In *The Lure of the Modern: Writing Modernism in Semicolonial China, 1917–1937,* Shu-mei Shih argues that the time of nation building where two world views met was envisioned by many of those participating in the process as a single trajectory. She argues that for Chinese modernists at that time, the trajectory of progress was a single, shared trajectory, where the only difference between East and West was time, and "not anything essential."[63] This melding of difference into one cosmopolitan and modernist developmental trajectory is explicitly rejected by present-day historical and post-development analysis, where ontological difference is at the heart of our interest and concern as scholars. Doreen Massey critiques such single teleologies, calling them a "historical queue," where difference in places around the world are collapsed into temporal differences on the pathway to a single modernity.[64] Yet for Shih, modernity has been discursively constructed as "occidental" or Western, when there is plenty of evidence for the role of Chinese thought in defining and implementing modernities that are in conversation and response to Western modernity but that are not necessarily Western themselves. Shih's work deals with literature, but I think here we get to the heart of the interactions between Chinese traditional medicine—*zhongyi*—and Western biomedicine—*xiyi*. In some ways, we can see *xiyi* as partly a discursive construction of China used by various groups to make points about China's need to catch up, or used in comparison to the strengths of *zhongyi*. For nurse Zhang, the two systems are not exactly integrated, but both are present and can be called on as needed.

The final point in this analysis of the engagements between *zhongyi* and *xiyi* is the emergence of the formalized practice of TCM, a state-supported and -regulated form of *zhongyi*. This regulated and formalized practice is partly a response to the need for mass primary health care instituted in the 1950s, but also, as Elisabeth Hsu has argued, "invented . . . during a period of nationalism marked by idealism and pride in China's ancient philosophy and cultural heritage." The formalization of TCM has made it more widely transmissible via classes and textbooks rather than the traditional mechanism of apprenticeship that was used for many thousands of years. This transmissibility was essential in the training of the "barefoot doctors" who drew on both Western and Chinese medical traditions and administered one of the most successful rural primary health care systems at the time, which included preventative health care like hygiene education and family planning. The use of an increasingly standardized TCM helped smooth the way for Western biomedicine in rural areas, according to Sanchun Xu and Danian Hu.[65] In many ways, this remade version of TCM has strived for integration into the ontology that Western modernity had proposed: the one-world world of science, where what is real is what is measurable and observable through the practices of science. Scholars have argued this is why TCM has emphasized its successful pharmacology and has subjected itself to the diagnostics of *xiyi,* as required by China's integrated health care system. Yet this formalized and integrated TCM creates space for something that is not the one-world world to shelter in its corridors and waiting rooms and in the homes of ordinary people concocting soups to promote the flow of blood, qi, and breast milk, or dressing children to prevent what is known as wind damage.[66]

How should we think about this multiplicity? How do we understand these multiple trajectories assembling in place to produce something— modernity, solid scientific ontologies, a one-world world, but also a shadow or ghost of something else? Before we get to that final point, allow me to introduce just one more trajectory into the mix as a way to understand how to engage in this kind of thinking. Here I turn to Eve Sedgwick's question in her book *Tendencies,* where she grasps at a scholarship that does not look only to confirm large patterns and constellations but also looks to the ghosts, the disjunctures, and the things that do not simply confirm what we already know. She asks, in a question that has echoed in my mind ever since I first read it, "What if the richest junctures weren't the ones where everything means the same thing?"[67]

SHADOW TRAJECTORIES

The story of hygienic modernity, integration, nation building, and formalization is compelling. Ruth Rogaski's work has shown how the term *weisheng* changed in meaning over the years to become a core component of nation building and public health as well as of conceptions of what it means to be modern in twentieth-century China. This Foucauldian-style biopolitics of the body, colonial thinking, nation-states, and imperialism is compelling, and indeed, it is often a story I tell in my first-year geography lectures on politics and place. However, it is not the only story, and it is certainly not the only trajectory for the concept of *weisheng.* This is important because in the nation-building stories of public health and hygiene, we can miss things. Sometimes these things are the very things we might need to build different kinds of future hygienes that are less about universals of hygiene and more about building hygiene communities that honor human health and the health of the planet. In what follows, I use Sean Hsiang-lin Lei's work to trace a ghost of a different kind of hygiene assembled momentarily in place in the republican era of Chinese history—a ghost of hygiene that might offer something novel about how social change happens and might help us explore the kinds of multiplicities created in any intersection of trajectories in place. It is a ghost that is also present in the hygiene assemblages of Xining in the twenty-first century, traceable in the interviews with women discussing their bodies and the bodies of their infants as they care for health in place.

Let me begin with Nie Yuntai. For many years, Nie Yuntai, a reformist, was a vocal campaigner for Western-style health and hygiene practices. He was a Christian and a wealthy industrialist who supported the ways of the West for much of his early life, including the need for Chinese families to adopt the hygiene practices of the Western- and Japanese-trained doctors who supported hygienic modernity in the post–Manchurian plague era. However, later in life, he converted to Buddhism, gave up his bathtub and his pursuit of hygienic modernity, and began critiquing the "morbid addiction to cleanliness" he saw around him.[68] Nie is said to have replaced his expensive bathroom fittings with a simple washbasin, in contrast to his previous efforts to convince the population of China's cities to adopt Western understandings of health and hygiene. After years of arguing that only through Western-style hygiene could China embrace modernity and kick the label of the "sick man of Asia" once and for all, why would Nie suddenly change his mind, and so drastically?

For Nie, the issue was not just whether hygienic modernity was effective in preserving health but also whether it was effective in establishing and maintaining the kind of community he wanted to be a part of. He concluded that the obsessive pursuit of "modern hygiene" was a sort of save-yourself-first individualism that could only be implemented by those with the material conditions to do so: the very wealthy. He argued that hygiene needed to be a set of simple practices that "could be implemented everywhere, including in places of poverty and simple homes."[69] He understood hygiene as being something intimately related not just to the functions and health of individual bodies but to the corporate body of society as a whole.

As Lei points out, Nie's vision of hygiene was in line with the traditional understanding of *weisheng* (guarding life) and *yangshang* (nurturing life). Using the writings of Nie Yuntai and other republican-era writers, Lei rereads the history of hygiene for difference,[70] sketching the boundaries of an alternative hygiene, or *weisheng,* articulated in response and opposition to the hygienic modernity discourse. Working discursively, he lays out the boundaries of what he calls "Chinese-style hygiene" to refer to "the alternative and specifically Chinese forms of hygiene that had not been incorporated into (or that positioned themselves outside of) Western-style hygiene."[71] This is most clearly made visible in Nie Yuntai's rejection of the accoutrements and individualism necessary for Western-style hygiene and in his promotion of a simple hygiene that is centered around the welfare of the community and society of which one is a part.

The "Chinese-style hygiene" that Lei is outlining for us is thus not an unchanging feature of traditional Chinese culture but rather a product of a specific historical encounter with other realities in time and place. It involved an absorption of some elements of Western-style hygiene and germ theory; it even translated some traditional Confucian elements of moral wellbeing into "medical instructions with concrete health benefits."[72] It also involved a rejection of certain elements of Western-style hygiene and a reinforcement of elements of Chinese tradition that contributed to wellbeing at a whole-society and whole-person level. Lei examines the intersection between hygiene and community through a number of hygiene examples, such as the custom of eating together. In Chinese tradition, food is shared from central dishes on a table, with diners helping themselves with their chopsticks multiple times at each meal. Proponents of Western-style hygiene argued that this approach to eating transmitted tuberculosis, and followers of Western-style hygiene were urged to make sure they helped themselves to the dishes first.[73] Nie argued that these antisocial behaviors of the Western-style approach rendered it careless, even unhygienic, if one considered the health of the entire *shen* (body and psyche) or *sheng* (life) of a person and that person's community. Alluding to the associations of TCM, he argued that obsessive individualist hygiene practices were in fact pathological; they caused disease through acts of selfishness and anxious worry about health, which disrupt the flow of qi. In his view, the Western overemphasis on the material causes of illness and its neglect of the spiritual and psychological links to wellness could actually result in more health problems, even if one were able to avoid tuberculosis. In this way of thinking, caring for others is good for both you and the ones you care for, in addition to being connected to the subsequent health of society.

In addition to the discussion of Nie's life and work, Lei provides us with many other examples at the intersection between hygiene and community, including communal sleeping arrangements, bathing styles, spitting, fresh air, and nutrition. In a further article, Lei investigates a number of material solutions to hygiene problems, including the deliberate invention of the so-called hygienic table (a lazy Susan with serving utensils for each dish), which preserves the sociality of eating without transmitting germs.[74] Lei demonstrates that while these alternative thinkers accepted the role of microbes in physical hygiene, they also "spared no costs to emphasize the importance of 'governing the heart' and of 'mental hygiene,' even regarding these aspects as the special contribution of Chinese *weisheng*."[75]

What Lei calls Chinese-style hygiene emerges as a point of resistance to a hygienic modernity focused exclusively on microbes and their interactions with only the material body. It is part of a broader Buddhist critique of Western-style science, a topic of frequent debate in the 1920s and 1930s in China.[76] Lei's uncovering of a Chinese-style hygiene makes visible a ghost present in the word *weisheng*: the tradition of holistically guarding life. Lei's work to make this ghost visible is not an easy task, however, because what he is describing does not have its own "name"—that is, both the discourses of modern hygiene and Chinese-style hygiene use the word *weisheng* to name something. Lei writes:

> One major difficulty in the methodology of researching this history lies in the fact that these alternative and indigenous Chinese discourses on *weisheng*, since they failed to meet with the approval of scholars of public health, never received their own specific and exclusive name. Because they attempted to partake of the same name as the Western concept of hygiene, they embarked on an uncertain and treacherous path. Subsumed under the popular term *weisheng*, they may have succeeded in initiating local endeavors that had little in common with the Western notion of hygiene; on the other hand, it is more likely that they were pushed out to the fringes of Western-style hygiene, to the point of vanishing into invisibility, as a result of this semantic confusion. Furthermore, how can historians possibly ascertain whether a phenomenon that does not have its own name even really exists? And how should they refer to it?[77]

Lei's object of research, these "alternative forms of hygiene," are referred to within just two pages of his 2009 article with fourteen different terms: "phenomena," "phenomenon," "conceptions," "practices and ideas," "discourses," "terms," "alternative hygiene," "Chinese-style hygiene," "endeavors," "forms," "practice," "entity," "creation," and "product." It is almost as if none of the words quite captures the nature of hygiene. Is it primarily a practice? A way of thinking? A bodily habit? An enterprise of the state? I think Lei's main difficulty lies in the problem of having to grasp, map, and name a messy assemblage cohabiting with the assemblage gathering around Western biomedicine at the same time. Lei does not make visible his own politics of research in his English-language work. We do not know why he wants to grasp what is almost invisible, that which is "pushed to the fringes, to the point of vanishing."[78] Is he interested in better establishing the facts of the history of hygiene? Or is he interested in constructing a space for new forms of hygiene to be nurtured? The question thus becomes not what hygiene realities are out there (for there are many), but which ones are described and made more real.[79]

Whatever his aim, Lei describes, names, and thereby makes (more) real a Chinese-style hygiene. In doing so, we can say Lei's work effectively gathers a hygiene assemblage where another hygiene reality has become (more) possible. Through exploring the partial connections (and disconnections) of the definitions of *weisheng,* Lei gathers microbes, practices, the body, thoughts, emotions, desires, qi and air, lazy Susans and chopsticks, sleeping platforms and washbasins, the writings of public figures, and the practices of the masses. He names this gathering Chinese-style hygiene. In doing this, Lei is pushing at the bounds of the singularity of hygiene, implying not a plurality of hygienes that are separate and contained but rather a multiplicity of hygiene realities interacting and interconnecting. It is a vision of interacting, overlapping hygiene realities. In outlining this second Chinese-style hygiene, which is not TCM, *zhongyi,* or *xiyi,* Lei is in fact calling into being multiple (but interrelated) hygiene realities, which are overlapping and extending into each other. In engaging with this multiplicity, the researcher's role becomes something other than a fact finder, trying to discover if something without a name can really exist. The researcher is participating in enacting a reality where this something does exist.

One important implication for my argument, however, is that Lei's study shows us that the trajectory of *weisheng* as hygienic modernity could have gone another way. He gives us a picture of hygiene as an ephemeral and slippery assemblage (of practices, knowledges, materialities), haunted by multiple might-have-beens, actively evolving and changing in response to the contingencies of history, space, and the intentional actions of people. Another implication of his study is that researchers participate in making some hygiene realities more real. That is, Lei's gathering and naming of Chinese-style hygiene somehow gives it more solidity, makes it more of a viable option—not just historically but also currently. The very naming of Chinese-style hygiene calls it into being. No longer a vague haunting drifting around the fringes of history, *weisheng* is now given form—a ghost that is traceable, though still ephemeral and difficult to grasp.

Let me return momentarily to nurse Zhang and the shifting assemblages that meet in her body and workplace in Xining. What role does this alternative, Chinese-style hygiene of urban twentieth-century Shanghai offer us in our thinking around bodies in place, as well as the multiplicity of trajectories that occupy them—indeed, that constitute them? While this shadow trajectory might not necessarily be visible in Zhang's story, it does raise the possibility of shifting assemblages that occupy the same space as the dominant trajectories with high visibility. We could read the history of hygiene as the inevitable victory of science and progress, yet Lei's Chinese-style hygiene shows a different science of progress. In turn, we could read the history of hygiene as the inevitable dominance of colonization processes, yet Lei's Chinese-style hygiene shows us the complex processes of hybridity and negotiation between multiple ontologies. These shadow trajectories offer a way of thinking about the awkward engagement of universals producing multiple new assemblages and realities, some of which are highly visible in our histories and some which are not. The mapping of the hygiene assemblage in Xining is thus never quite complete.

A SHIFTED ASSEMBLAGE

The place of Xining and the "place closest in" to the bodies of Xining residents are collections of stories, specific "articulations within the wider power-geometries of space," as Doreen Massey puts it.[80] There is much more that could be said about the collections of stories and power geometries of Xining—of development, hygiene, medicine, and more. Much of rural Qinghai is home to a variety of different ethnic minorities (45 percent of the provincial population), while urban areas are dominated by ethnic Han people, the majority group in China. The city of Xining is around three-quarters Han. It was a migration destination during the early twentieth century as part of a push for national unity and ethnic intermingling, as well as a current migration destination for immigrants and investors from northeast China. The urban–rural divide in this part of the country is also partly an ethnic divide, with the culturally dominant Han shaping acceptable norms. Some of my participants showed a tendency to line up ethnic groups in terms of their quality and modernity. Indeed, some Hui Muslim participants spoke of their own feudalism and feudal backwardness compared to the Han.[81] For many, the historical queue–type analysis traceable in the trajectories of medicine and modernity mentioned earlier applied within the nation of China as well, where backward peoples needed to somehow catch up.

The caregiving practices of minorities and rural migrants in Xining were thus understood as somehow lacking, ignorant, low status, superstitious, and *ku*, "bitter." While each person in Qinghai has no doubt been affected by the multiple trajectories of health, hygiene, and bodies that have assembled in this part of China, the difference articulated between caregivers was not about different medical traditions but different socioeconomic positions, where what was modern and scientific in caregiving and hygiene was assumed to be the practices of wealthy Han and foreign families. Their practices were described as cultured, changing for the better, hygienic, and educated. This was mainly about discourse, as they were described in this way even if their practices were not in fact generally known or necessarily supported by published biomedical research (for example, the middle-class practice of educating babies in the womb known as *taijiao*).[82] The shape of the hygiene assemblage in Xining in the early 2000s, then, is a result of the dynamic simultaneity of historical and contemporary trajectories gathered in place, some of which I have traced in this chapter. The hygiene assemblage—which includes the specific practice of baniao and some of the social, spatial, historical, and material context of the practice—cannot be transported to anywhere else in the world. Yet certain elements of this assemblage, particularly the practice of infant toileting, have traveled to other parts of Australia and New Zealand, partly through my own accidental interventions.

Situated Hygienes

Summer 2007. Xining, China. My first child, clothed in split-crotch pants and sturdy sandals, is squatting outdoors in our *xiaoqu* exercise area, examining ants. She tires of squatting and plonks her bare bottom on the concrete. I automatically reach over and pull her to her feet, supporting her in a squat so she can continue her study. It is not that I am worried about her bare bottom being in contact with concrete, although that cannot be too comfortable. It is more that I just know she should not do that here, just as I know she must always wear shoes and shirts with sleeves. How do I know this? In 2007, I do not even know I know this, but I do it nonetheless. My body knows it.

Winter 2011. Bankstown, Sydney, Australia. My toddler is toddling around barefoot on the concrete area outside the school hall, where inside, her five-year-old sister has just performed in the school production. She toddles, wobbles, then plonks down hard on the concrete, fortunately protected by her cloth nappy, waterproof cover, and stretchy leggings. Refusing my outstretched hand and its offer to help her regain her feet, she crawls across the concrete and pulls herself up on the brick wall to begin again. Midway through the next cycle she stops, looks at me, and says "unh."

"Do you need to go potty?" I ask.

She looks around for a potty, which I take as a yes. Unfortunately, the toilet is inside the crowded school hall, and I would have to push through other parents watching the performance to get there. I make a quick decision. I pick her up and walk around behind the building. Looking around to see if anyone can see me, I quickly pull down her leggings and remove her nappy, holding her out on the grass. She immediately urinates, and with some difficulty, I manage to put her nappy back on with her balanced on my knee. The tension goes out of my shoulders as the operation is completed without having to explain myself to anyone.

Winter 2014. Christchurch, New Zealand. My nine-month-old is clothed in a thick cloth nappy and warm onesie pajamas. We have all the doors closed to the lounge room of our small, carpeted, uninsulated rental home, and the heater is on high. I glance at my watch and realize it is evening potty time. I get out a box of wooden toy blocks and set up the white plastic potty on the lounge room floor. I lay him down on the carpet, undo his pajamas, remove his nappy, then lift him onto the potty. He immediately grabs for the bricks, and I set my older daughters (now eight and four years old) the task of building towers for him to knock down as he gets his evening poop out of the way.

Early autumn 2019. Christchurch, New Zealand. My three-month-old is having his midmorning breastfeed while I read a proof copy of a book chapter on my smartphone. My parental leave is finished, but I have some sabbatical time to work on an edited book. He pulls away from my breast and then tries to latch back on. I put down my phone and use my hand to guide the breast back into his mouth. I pick up the phone to read the next page. He pulls off again, pulling his knees up to his chest. I pick him up over my shoulder and do up my bra, calling my husband as I do so. My husband emerges from the kitchen, and I hand him the baby.

"Output time!" I say.

We joke that I am the "input manager" and he is the "output manager" for our fourth child. I am working full time, breastfeeding night and day, while he is in his tenth year as the official stay-at-home parent. He grabs the small plastic bucket we have been using as a potty and holds out the baby in a cradle hold. I return to my work as a small, yellow arc narrowly misses the bucket and partly ends up on the wooden floors. My husband drops a muslin cloth onto the puddle, and the baby releases some loud gas. Nothing else emerges, and my husband readjusts the newborn-size split-crotch pants and wraps the baby in a light blanket, lifting him onto his shoulder to burp. He wipes the floor with his foot, then carries the bucket and cloth one-handed to the laundry sink at the back of the house. I hear him run water as I go out the back door into the sunshine with the baby, ready to flip open my laptop to write up the chapter corrections.

We are old hands these days, at both parenting and infant toileting. Now, after buying a run-down rental, we had the means to adjust our home to a hybrid baniao environment. We knocked out walls to create an open-plan, sunny living area; we stripped the floors back to the original wood; and we insulated the walls, ceiling, and floor. One of my PhD students, from Qinghai, brought over a selection of cotton split-crotch infant cloth-ing—we had given our baby stuff away years ago. Another friend gifted us her collection of traditional flat cloth nappies used for many of her four children. The paraphernalia of infant toileting included a new mop and an upgraded washing machine. We bought our first dryer. We dug out old clothes, potties, and buckets from the garage. I rejoined an online group for infant toileting (or elimination communication), this time on Facebook. The assemblage of hygiene I found gathered here was material, social, spa-tial, and economic. It was also situated in time and place. It is no longer unusual to practice infant toileting—a cultural shift that has happened in the thirteen years since we had our first child.

4 Traveling Practices

> Perhaps people are starting to see the madness of our
> disposable nappy driven, four-year-olds-in-nappies society
> and we're the beginning of a move back towards early
> [toilet training] as the norm.
> —Ainslie, 2008

> Well, I figured if kids in [other countries] can be toilet
> trained by 12 months, my kids aren't any more stupid than
> any of theirs.
> —Nadine, 2009

Despite the ubiquity of baniao-type practices globally, they are currently familiar to only a minority of parents in Western nations such as Australia and New Zealand. In the context of late toilet training, landfill pressures, and concerns about the environmental impact of both disposable and cloth nappies, these practices merit exploration. In this chapter, I make visible the shifting and experimental hybrid hygiene assemblage of Australian and New Zealand practitioners of the baniao-like practice of elimination communication. I use this experimental assemblage to begin thinking about how changes in care practices can happen through this gathering of new hygiene assemblages, a theme taken up in more detail in chapter 5.

My embodied experience in practicing EC and baniao with my own four children certainly informs this chapter in many ways. However, in order to get a sense of the wider assemblage of hygiene in which I am embedded and implicated, this chapter is based mainly on material gathered from OzNappyfree, the online nappy-free support forum I was a member of for more than ten years. OzNappyfree is a Yahoo! Group of, at one time, more than five hundred mothers, based mostly in Australia and New Zealand, who supported each other in learning and practicing EC. While most of this activity has now shifted to Facebook, my analysis of the forum is a timely reminder of the way technologies shape and change our communication practices as well as our care and hygiene practices.

Using ethnographic material from this web forum, in this chapter I describe the practice of EC in its Australian and New Zealand context, focusing particularly on how practitioners are rejecting the idea that developed places are necessarily more advanced than less-developed contexts when it comes to health and hygiene. I mainly use the detailed web posts of EC parents on OzNappyfree, supplemented with two focus groups in Melbourne and Brisbane and observations at a Sydney meet-up. I include some brief observations gleaned from later research featuring Facebook groups for EC in Australia and New Zealand. In the last section of the chapter, I show how EC parents situated their practice within a global diversity of toileting and parenting techniques that fall outside what is considered mainstream in their own societies. Drawing on these contemporaneous "other modernities" challenges teleological understandings of care practices, hygiene, and modernity, thus providing a gap for these parents to experiment with alternative forms of hygiene keeping. This can be thought of as a form of direct activism, where mothers and others work toward change for a better world in a number of key areas, including infant emotional development, ecoconsciousness, circular economies, and water-use reduction. I finish the chapter with some thoughts on the changes in hygiene assemblages, social media, and environmental parenting in the decade since these data were collected.

The locally enacted universal baby's bottom of baniao and similar practices has global significance. Further, it is a bridge by which the practice of infant toileting is traveling and new hybrid assemblages of hygiene are being gathered in places as far away as Australia. The infant body in these Western places is no longer bound by the facts recorded in Western experience and science. Rather, through the very knowledge of other alternatives, it becomes a different kind of body multiple. In this case, it awakens multiple possible embodied realities of muscle control, (pre)cognition, and infant hygiene, with ongoing implications for hygiene and care practices around the world. While a baniao form of infant hygiene care is time-consuming and ostensibly inconvenient, it is understood to be part of being in a family and caring for a baby's health. In the next chapter, we examine how this is extended into Australian and New Zealand care assemblages, multiplying the possible embodied realities of infants, adopted as a way of caring for the infant–caregiver relationship and the environment, with a good dose of anticorporate affect thrown in.

HYGIENE ALTERNATIVES

Variously referred to as infant pottying, natural infant hygiene, diaper/nappy-free babies, early toileting, and elimination communication, the practice of holding out babies to eliminate their waste occasionally makes the news in Western nations. Various parenting magazines have featured the practice, such as Claire Sibonney's detailed article, "Elimination Communication," in *Today's Parent*. A mother rose to TikTok fame in 2022 after her baby toileting posts went viral, according to a *New Zealand Herald* article.[1] The *Guardian*'s lifestyle and parenting section has featured the practice.[2] Mayim Bialik, an American actress known for her work on the hit TV show *The Big Bang Theory*, has spoken about EC with her two children.[3] I myself first heard of nappy-free babies via a friend in the United Kingdom, who had seen a newspaper article there in 2005. Typically, media reports on EC oppose the practice to widespread delayed toilet training, playing the medical community against EC parents by placing quotes from nurses or pediatricians (who say EC is unlikely to be anything but parent training) alongside interviews with parents describing their child's toileting successes in glowing terms. Emily Dunn, for example, frames her report in *Sydney Morning Herald* in terms of "who should decide when to toilet train—you or your baby?," thereby categorizing EC as a more parent-driven approach as well as a backlash against ever-later toilet training milestones.[4]

Dunn's article appears to be largely in response to a non-peer-reviewed report released by University of New South Wales researcher Anna Christie, who is disgusted by the way in which Australian parents appear to have "abandoned" toilet training.[5] This report mentions EC as an emerging fringe movement among tertiary-educated Australian mothers that skews the data. If ECers are not taken into account, mothers with higher education in her study were more likely than their less-educated counterparts to delay toilet training and less likely to offer assistance or direction in their children's toileting (unless asked directly by their children).[6] Regarding current toilet training practices in this group of more-educated mothers,

Christie writes, "Mothers tended to wait for verbal signs of [toilet training] readiness, but were not attuned to non-verbal or pre-verbal cues."[7] While many parents "believe they are toilet training," Christie opines in regard to the "child-centered" approach to toilet training readiness, "all they have done is remove the nappies and . . . offer some directions to the child."[8] In recent years, smartphone access to the internet enables parents to access toilet training advice from anywhere, ranging from official sources like the national ministry of health and the Mayo Clinic to TikTok and YouTube parenting channels. Facebook parenting groups have proliferated, and rapid toilet training methods are also making a comeback. Members of the group that I researched in 2009 all had access to the internet and many sources of information, but unlike today, they did not have smartphones. Instead, people usually accessed the internet through a laptop or desktop computer. This meant that they usually sat down intentionally, when their children were doing something else, such as sleeping.[9] This slow approach to internet use is somewhat different than today's instant access, and it shaped the way information was researched and shared.

The group of EC practitioners on whom I base my research communicated virtually through a Yahoo! Group known as OzNappyfree. Yahoo! Groups, a service provided by Yahoo! from 2001 to 2020, were a popular way to connect with others on topics of interest in the mid-2000s. People could sign onto forums of interest and receive (and reply to) posts by email, or they could choose to log on to the forums to scroll through previous posts. Posts were organized into threads around topics within the group, with etiquette norms normalized whereby if a discussion morphed into a new topic, a moderator or other member would start a new thread with the topic in the header. For those accessing the posts mainly via email, this would appear as an email thread with the previous replies listed below, much like a Reply All email in the workplace today.

OzNappyfree was set up in 2004 by Sydney IT analyst Marnie Holmes. It was an offshoot of the North American Diaperfree Yahoo! Group. Marnie remained a member of the North American group but thought that ECers Down Under needed a space to discuss EC that was relevant to their experiences. She considered the main differences to be due to climate and the opposite seasons (for example, discussions on what to wear for EC in the winter were always coming up during the Australian summer), as well of course the obvious linguistic differences of British English "nappy" versus American English "diaper."

The parents who participated in OzNappyfree mostly came from a fairly educated background and favored a child-centered or attachment-parenting approach including practices such as cosleeping (sharing a bed with children), baby wearing (carrying babies around in slings or soft carriers for most of the day), breastfeeding on demand for a relatively extended period, and gentle or positive discipline (nonpunitive). For many of these parents, EC simply extended the child-centered approach into the area of toilet learning, where the baby's signals and cues for elimination are taken as the starting point for toilet opportunities from birth rather than waiting until the age of verbal communication to begin the process. For others in the group, EC came first and led to these other attachment-parenting practices, which fit well with the nonverbal and trust-based communication approach of EC.

I collected web-post content (with permission from group members and Marnie) throughout 2009. By the end of that year, the group had 453 members, although in December 2009, a total of thirty-five mothers contributed 100 percent of the posts. Members posted questions, advice, and reflections on EC practice and strategies, along with regular off-topic discussions, prefaced in the subject line as "OT." These OT discussions grew more and more frequent during 2008 as a core group of members came to rely on each other for advice in all kinds of parenting-related areas—to the point that Marnie set up a secondary group for other parenting discussions of ECing parents. This group grew to a membership of around forty mothers, who regularly posted until around 2014, with many having gone on to have subsequent children. I have included both groups in my 2009 content analysis, since in the OT group the ECers often reflect on the wider effects of EC in their parenting styles and in the community. In 2015, I invited all members of OzNappyfree to write a reflection on their last few years (since 2009) and on the ways EC had affected their other parenting and hygiene practices. From 2013 to 2017, I also followed the Elimination Communication in Australia Facebook group, which is the Facebook presence of OzNappyfree.

The infant toileting practices of the families in Australia and New Zealand had some overlap with those in northwest China, but they also had many differences. For the most part, the cultural and spatial context was unsupportive of infant toileting, so mainly people who felt strongly about the social and environmental benefits pursued the practice. However, in detailing the practices as follows, it becomes clear that the cultural and spatial knowledges for non-Western cultures and places were important in the development of the practice in Australia and New Zealand.

STARTING OUT

OzNappyfree members sometimes joined the group before their babies were born. Some heard about the group from other forums in Australia and New Zealand or through meeting a member at a playgroup. When new people signed up for OzNappyfree, they received an email asking them about themselves, their children (and their ages), their EC experience, where they lived, where they heard about the group, and whether they belonged to any other EC groups. Once this email was returned, forum moderator Marnie approved their membership in the group, and they were able to start reading posts, receiving posts as emails, and posting questions via the Yahoo! Group or directly via email. Most often, pregnant and new members asked to hear others' experiences of ECing immediately after birth, be it in hospital or home.

While some learned how to EC by asking direct questions, others browsed the Australian website Tribal Baby or read one of the books available on EC, most often Australian doctor Sarah J. Buckley's *Gentle Birth, Gentle Mothering,* which describes EC in one of the chapters. Other common books mentioned were those by Ingrid Bauer and Laurie Boucke, and more recently Andrea Olson.[10] These resources emphasize the "gentle" aspect of EC, deliberately distancing themselves from earlier disciplinarian forms of early toilet training in the West. These books are all written by mothers practicing EC, and all refer mostly to full-time EC, whereby the primary caregiver attempts to go almost completely without any reliance on nappies, remaining ever vigilant to elimination communications from their baby.

In preparation for EC, forum members have variously suggested the following purchases: a bowl, basin, or tiny potty for catching eliminations; cloth nappies with no covers so as to easily feel when the child is wet; easily removable clothing (no all-in-one suits); and plastic-backed mats or lanolinized woolen blankets[11] to protect surfaces from accidents. Those who planned to EC full time sometimes avoided many of the standard pregnancy purchases, including forgoing bassinets and baby beds for the close contact of cosleeping/bed sharing; forgoing infant seats, prams, or strollers; and swapping structured carriers for soft slings. A number of the mothers from OzNappyfree ran small "mumpreneur" businesses importing, making, and selling EC equipment, books, and DVDs.[12]

NEWBORN AND IN-ARMS STAGE

Although some members reported holding out their babies within hours of birth, many members started with a period of observation, where the baby was kept nappy-free for a set period of time each day as the family tried to observe any signs that precede elimination. Newborn signs include passing gas, making a "pushing" face, drawing up the knees repeatedly, fussing at the breast, crying and squirming, suddenly increasing motion such as rapid arm waving or leg kicking, or suddenly ceasing motion. Other newborns simply eliminate every time they breastfeed, so mothers sometimes breastfed babies seated on a flat nappy or over a small potty held between the knees.

First-catch stories were a common way to introduce oneself to the group, often containing a lot of detail explaining when and how the catcher knew to hold out the baby. Tamara wrote the following, showing her joy and pleasure in that first catch:

> Well I didn't think I'd be writing so soon with success but . . . Our little boy Evan is just over 3 weeks now. This morning I caught our first poos and wees in the potty and the toilet!!! I was so thrilled it was as much as I could do not to wake my sleeping husband and share the good news!!! I had Evan on the change mat about to change between sides as I was bfeeding . . . when he started to "push" as he does so clearly. I also needed the loo (!) I took him with me and sat on the loo with him . . . I had him with his back up against my tummy and opened my legs wide enough so that his bum had room to get in there . . . said the magic word, caca (we use) and ssss . . . and sure enough he started pooing. (web post, August 2009)

Tamara describes what is known as the classic position, where the baby is held in a squat-like position over a receptacle, with the back against the adult's stomach or leaning on the adult's forearms, knees higher than bottom. This is the position referred to as *baniao* in Mandarin Chinese. The second common position is the cradle or reclined position, where the newborn baby is held reclined on one forearm as if being rocked, with both the adult's hands grasping under the thighs, directing the bottom toward the receptacle—the advantage of this position for newborns being that their head is supported (Figure 6). Both positions serve to straighten out the sphincter and allow the release of any eliminations. In the early days, babies eliminate almost every time they are held in one of the two common EC positions. The elimination is then reinforced with a cue—sometimes a low whistle, as described earlier, but often a sibilant, water sound such as "ssss" or "shhh" as they urinate, or a grunt or cue word such as "poo-poo" as they defecate.

As the baby comes to associate the release of the sphincter muscle with the cue word and position, the cue word soon becomes a prompt to release rather than merely a comment on it. The ability to relax and release the muscle is the first stage of EC learning for the baby, and even from this early age, the process quickly becomes much more interactive than merely timing and catching. It is not uncommon for babies in the early days to be dry through the night if they are consistently offered the potty when waking to feed. Some members explained this through reference to published medical research: if a baby went down dry and cycled through the first REM sleep cycle and then into quiet sleep before waking, the baby would often stay dry because babies rarely eliminate during quiet sleep.[13]

Many of the babies still wore nappies much of the time. Summer and tropical babies spent some of the day dressed in a top layer only; they were carried around with a cloth nappy or towel underneath them. Winter babies were sometimes dressed in warm nightgowns and booties with a nappy

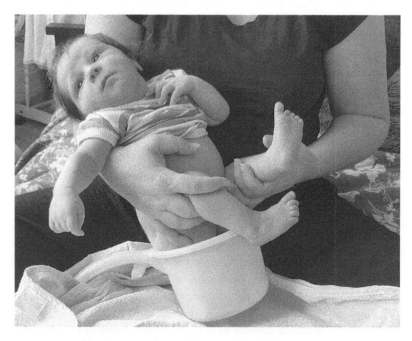

FIGURE 6. Holding out a newborn. Photograph by Travis Dombroski, 2019.

underneath them, then wrapped in a blanket or carried in a sling. Part-time ECers, who were by far the most numerous, tended to fully dress their babies and use nappies either with or without covers. They then offered "pottytunities" (potty opportunities) when changing nappies, or they simply removed the entire bottom half of clothing as needed.

At this stage, there were few messy misses—or at least no more than conventionally nappied babies who spend some time each day "having a kick" (lying on the floor with no nappy on, normally on a towel or mat). The major issue reported during this period of EC is the interactions with family members and health professionals. First-time parents especially reported feeling embarrassed about the whole thing, even trying to hide it from relatives and medical staff for fear of scorn. One ECer wrote, "Although supportive, even my mother thinks that I am making extra work for myself." In the Brisbane focus group, Nadine thought that EC had isolated her from seeking help from family and health professionals because of the feeling of surveillance:

> I think this feeling of being watched, that you're being watched by a bunch of people who want you to fail and this sounds like I think everyone's horrible, I don't, but I think its just natural that when you're struggling, everyone's struggling with mothering, they are all struggling with guilt, they are all struggling with the fact that their mother or their husband or their husband's father doesn't necessarily agree with what they are doing in a multitude of areas, and then to take upon yourself another area where everyone disagrees with you! From the start and you just have to push, push, push through and just in a way, by committing to do it, you are committing to not talk to anyone about it. Because they get upset and they get vindictive and they get angry—and it can be quite isolating.

ECers' fears of health professionals and family members seemed to be more common than actual reported negative interactions. Although these incidents were uncommon, they served to feed the fear of being watched—a sense expressed by a number of first-time mothers on the forum before they gained confidence in their parenting style and caregiving practices.

MOBILE BABIES

As babies grew and changed, so did EC practice. The signs of imminent elimination often became less clear as new frustrations were introduced into the babies' lives beyond hunger, discomfort, and tiredness. Some big milestones began occurring around six months, including increasing mobility, introduction of solids, and increasing ability to communicate and eliminate more consciously.

Once the baby could sit, many of the ECers started relying on the use of potties and seat reducers on the toilet. Babies were then dressed in easy-to-remove pants with nappies or training pants (padded underwear that absorbs one miss), some wearing split-crotch pants in the Chinese style, some wearing ingenious drop-flap nappies. A few left their babies bare bottomed, with leg warmers and a long top worn in cooler weather. Clothing at this age depended not only on the weather but also the house: those families living in carpeted rental houses in cooler climates were the most likely to keep their babies fully nappied once they were mobile. Mobility also could become tricky for ECers that used potties (rather than holding out), who found that their babies could get off the potty before having finished (or even started) their eliminations. Distraction with books, toys, or games became important while waiting for the baby to relax the appropriate muscles. Dave wrote of his ten-month-old:

> Giving her a toy or reading her a book really helps her settle for long enough to relax and let the wee out (otherwise she just stands straight up and jumps off the potty). (web post, March 2009)

ECers who held out their baby also sometimes found resistance to the elimination position, even if the baby clearly needed to eliminate, often because the baby was interested in doing something other than toileting. Many members reported potty pauses during this stage, where they go from high to low catch rates, often within a few weeks. Some returned to full-time nappy use and stopped offering pottytunities regularly, while others continued to offer pottytunities when they spotted a sign, or at certain times of the day, until the baby adjusted. Dave again:

> Offering pottytunities is harder these days because she is such a squirmer to get the nappy and clothes back on (need to move to Queensland where its warmer!), so it would be good to reinforce the signalling. I've been thinking of easing back on the timing-based offers and wait more for signals. (web post, March 2009)

A second factor contributing to changes in EC practice was the introduction of solids. Current recommendations in Australia and New Zealand were, and remain, to begin introducing solids around six months, when certain signs of readiness are exhibited, and no earlier than four months. The World Health Organization's recommendation was six months at the earliest, and most ECers followed this as a rule of thumb. Many of the OzNappyfree members followed a method of introducing solids known as baby-led weaning, which prioritizes breastfeeding as the main source of nutrition for the first year, with babies encouraged to feed themselves with finger foods from six months. Once solids were introduced, the baby's digestive system changes, normally leading to less frequent and more solid feces, which the baby must consciously excrete. Holding the baby in the classic position helped this excretion process but would no longer necessarily prompt it. At this stage, some people also reported that their babies rarely defecated while out of the home, preferring to wait until home to defecate in their own potty or over their own toilet.

The introduction of solids also affected EC in other ways. ECers were well positioned to notice any food sensitivities in their children. For babies with food sensitivities, the first sign of intolerance was an obvious increase in urine frequency and volume after certain foods, or greenish-colored feces or diarrhea. Common food sensitivities that caused obvious changes in urine frequency were dairy, wheat, certain preservatives, and amine-, sulfur-, and salicylate-containing foods. Kristina reported:

> Foods that I have noticed increase wees for us are: melons, grapes, citrus. Too much tomato-based things. I try to rotate the tomato-based foods so there are a couple of days with none . . . and I realise we have slipped a bit with the diet, as there are a few things that are needing attention such as light sleeping. I do feel that it makes a difference for us with her awareness about wees. No surprise wees/misses. (web post, June 2009)

Some babies grew out of these early sensitivities by the time they got to the mainstream toilet training age of two and did not go on to have food sensitivities.[14]

A third factor contributing to changes in EC practice is babies' increasing ability to consciously communicate and eliminate. Communication can take the form of verbal noises and the beginnings of words, sign language, or other deliberate signals, and movement such as tapping the potty or moving toward the bathroom. Several OzNappyfree members signed with their babies from around seven months of age, teaching their babies how to use Australian or New Zealand Sign Language to sign "potty," "toilet," "wee-wee," or "poo-poo," as well as other signs such as "milk," "hurting," and "drink." Babies from this age were capable of signing preemptively, although more often they used the sign after the fact of elimination to signal that they had gone.

As babies developed the ability to "hold on," EC became much more about getting the baby to relax and release when they showed signs of needing to go. The creativity of EC parents at this stage was crucial; they came up with all sorts of interesting methods to help their babies relax and eliminate. ECers began to find that their babies were willing to urinate into one potty and not another, in one room but not another, in one position but not another, and even with one person present and not another. The web forum archive has hundreds of posts offering suggestions on helping babies during this stage. If ECers know the baby needs to go, they could begin with the cue sounds developed earlier, then try various positions, rooms, and potties; they could try reading stories, singing songs, taking deep, relaxing breaths (which the baby copies), running water—anything to get the baby to relax and eliminate. This stage appears to be the most time-consuming and difficult stage of the EC journey, and many ECers backed off the whole process at this point. Yet looking at the monthly updates posted for ECers with babies in this stage, most were still catching 95 percent of bowel movements and reported feeling pleased about not having to clean these up, even if urine misses were frequent.

For those having difficulty reading baby's signs yet not willing to give up and go back to full-time nappies, timing became their main method of catching their baby's eliminations. Some ECers were rather scientific about this; they would observe and record the times of day their baby eliminated, along with other important factors such as drinks, feeds, sleeps, and outings. They then offered their baby pottytunities when the baby was most likely to go—for example, at twenty and forty minutes after a drink. Others developed a sense of intuition around the timing of eliminations, offering when they intuited the baby needed to go based on absorbing patterns of elimination as much as signs or signals from the baby. Some ECers reported an 80 percent catch rate based on timing alone. Some parents prioritized catches over independence, taking responsibility for their child's body as a sort of extension of their own. Amber, who identified herself as an Australian-born Chinese woman with four children, wrote in this vein:

> Overall our parenting style is NOT to push them towards independence, we tend to follow a more Asian style of doing a lot for them, so others may have different desires and aims. I guess I am also a more controlling type of person in general, and I really don't like accidents, so I did try to push for potty perfection as well as communication, again other people may have differing styles and goals. (web post, November 2009)

Others preferred to leave the process more up to their child's communication style and had stronger ideals regarding children's right to control their own bodies. Indeed, this is in line with current Western toilet training models, which places the onus on children to toilet train as soon as they are ready and willing. Members with this latter approach who continued with EC during potty pauses had higher tolerance and acceptance of accidents. One New Zealand–based member spent her entire EC journey with her youngest son defecating daily on the laundry floor; he disliked pooing in nappies and wanted to poo standing up rather than in a potty or toilet. Kimberly, a mother of a six-month-old baby, wrote of accidents during this stage:

> I seem to be getting much more of a feeling for when he needs to wee and am more alert to his signs/signals since I have been leaving nappies off during awake time at home. In spite of the messy misses I have tried to just clean up and continue on. I'm glad that when there have been messes it has never been anywhere near as terrible as my imagination had led me to believe. Getting peed and poo'ed on isn't as terrible as I thought it was. (web post, November 2009)

The age of emerging mobility and communication, along with a changing diet, heralded a transition to a more concentrated EC effort. This was the most common stage under discussion on OzNappyfree, and the forum was an important part of ECers' lives as they sought guidance and inspiration from other ECers online.

TODDLERS TO TOILET TRAINERS

Because ECers envisioned the whole journey as a toilet-learning process rather than a toilet training process, the culmination of the journey is normally referred to as graduation—that is, children graduate from toilet learning and go on to toileting independence. The final year of EC, from around fifteen months until graduation, was a stage of constant renegotiation and of handing over increasing responsibility for toileting awareness to the child. During this period, the differences between full-time and part-time ECers became more apparent, as full-time ECers seemed to graduate much earlier into dryness (as early as nine months, through to around twenty-four months), with part-time ECers varying wildly from early graduation to rather late, even compared to conventionally trained children.

During the latter stages of EC, there was great variation in the use of potties, toilets, and holding out and in the types of clothing, nappies, trainers, and undies that were used. There were also several ECers who changed their approach from one of elimination communication to one of overt toilet training by using sticker charts, drill methods, and promises of big-kid undies and other rewards. The different approaches between those who offered based on the adult's timing, intuition, or schedule (offerers) and those who waited for signals from the baby (waiters) became more apparent here too. For those accustomed to offering on the adult's terms, there had to be a transition between relying on offering and timing to relying on the child's own ability to communicate a desire to eliminate, and finally the child's own ability to get to an appropriate toileting spot and remove clothing independently.

Elizabeth, a mother of a twenty-two-month-old who was part-time ECed, posted asking for "tips for encouraging DS to tell me beforehand" (where DS is internet shorthand for "dear/darling son"). She related her child's almost "100% poo miss rate" (in nappies or trainers) over the previous few months. She got a variety of responses, with Janelle suggesting teaching him baby signing, myself wondering whether it was easier to teach him where to go rather than expect him to lead, Annette suggesting he might want more independence or privacy, Dina suggesting putting the potty in the shower recess if he wanted privacy, and Rebecca suggesting signing and reinforcing every instance of his signing "potty" with a trip to the potty even if he did not need to go right then and was just copying the sign. This led to another discussion started by Rebecca, with the subject line "Offering vs. them asking & a graduation question." Rebecca wrote regarding her twenty-one-month-old:

Now my thoughts were that you should encourage them to ask for the toilet, once they get to a certain age, and certainly by the 18-month mark. I don't want to be pre-empting all his wees/poos when he is at an age when can tell me. So Kate's viewpoint made me stop and think. . . . I don't wait for DS to tell me he's hungry before I feed him, I pre-empt that, so why is the toileting any different? . . . I know if I take him to the toilet he will wee pretty much every time, even if it's only half an hour after the last wee . . . [but then] how will he learn that really full bladder feeling, and what to do? And as for graduating . . . I guess this is why I am so interested in the offer vs. them asking thing. *If* I offered based on timing, I am quite sure DS would be dry, definitely while awake, and quite probably if I always took him before he went down for a nap . . . what are people's thoughts on this? (web post, November 2009).

The answering posts reveal a range of perspectives on the graduation issue. Some writers used the one hundred hours benchmark, meaning that graduation referred to one hundred hours of continuous dryness, no matter how that is achieved. For Amber's first daughter, this occurred at around fourteen months; according to Rebecca above, this would be entirely possible for her son if she chose to follow the offering route. Others agreed with Annette that graduation has occurred "when I can't remember the last time I worried about his toileting"—that is, a significant period of either complete toilet independence or complete reliability in communicating toileting needs to an adult.

Annette later posted wondering if EC had been a mistake because several of her friends' children had toilet trained overnight, without the years of EC and hassle that Annette had experienced (although she later posted that it was worth it for the number of cloth nappies saved). The concern with when graduation can be said to have happened, and the "offering by adults" versus "waiting for signals or child to ask" discussion, reflects an awkward engagement between EC ideas of a gentle journey of gradual toilet learning and conventional Western ideas of toilet training as an event or milestone that occurs sometime between the second and third birthday (or later). Worrying about the moment of toilet training completion probably occurs in a cultural context where parents are often asked whether their child is toilet trained or has begun toilet training. The concern surrounding whether toilet training occurs faster or earlier is one that reflects the pressure of ECers to prove that their method is better than conventional toilet training—where better means earlier, more reliable, and less hassle for the caregiver.

Lila, another part-time ECer, illustrates this awkward engagement when reporting her daughter's graduation from "EC to TT" (toilet trained). Generally a waiter rather than an offerer, she writes,

> at about 21 months I read some of . . . and had several discussions around "potty-training in 3 days" [a drill method of potty training used by people who need to rapidly toilet train]. A friend was (for medical reasons) trying to toilet train her very unaware (her words) son. Something clicked and I took DD's nappy off. Very rapidly things clicked for DD (or maybe she was waiting for me?) and we were nappy free at home, including day sleeps. (web post, August 2009)

Lila did not follow the three-day method; nor did she really instigate any training as such. However, discussions with her friend around issues in conventional toilet training alerted her to the fact that her daughter was actually highly aware of her eliminations. Lila relates how, each step of the way, she realized that it was she, not the infant, who needed to "take a deep breath" and remove nappies. After her daughter started coming up to her and signing toilet (rather than signing only to herself), Lila "was brave enough to send her [to daycare] without a nappy on, forcing them to toilet her." Lila summarized her EC journey as follows:

> I have tried to let DD guide me, but also needed to give her the environment in which she could learn and move forward, and to get over my own fear/ impatience of dealing with public accidents/dealing with potties/finding toilets/asking shop owners to use their toilets etc. . . . We have toilet trained slowly, at the end of a great EC journey that was filled with many many books, potty songs, and lots of fun. (web post, August 2009)

Amber, the aforementioned offerer, likewise related a positive graduation experience, with both her daughters out of nappies before their second birthdays, the older one at fourteen months. In response to concerns that relying on offering might delay the child's development of their own awareness of a full bladder and toileting needs, Amber wrote that although she was still using a lot of timing and offering when she announced that her second daughter had graduated at twenty-two months, since that time (about three weeks), her daughter had "gone to telling me fully when she needs to pee/poo, or simply taken herself to the potty and peed herself without me knowing." All this had apparently "happened on her own steam," without Amber pushing her to be independent in any way because "basically they do it when they are ready."[15]

As in China, EC does not stop at graduation but continues for years, as various children still rely on their parents to manage certain aspects of toileting, such as washing hands, removing clothing, and finding public toilets. Annette compared practicing EC to swimming lessons: the point of taking a six-month-old to swimming lessons is not to get them swimming independently but to start them on a positive journey of increasing water confidence. The point here is that EC is a journey of communication rather than a task-focused toilet training program, and ECers and their babies displayed considerable variation in their approaches to managing this communication.

GLOBAL NORMS

OzNappyfree members imagine their practice of EC as part of the global norm for infant hygiene. Because baniao is a contemporaneous practice common throughout China, and because it is holding out (pun intended) against the aggressive marketing practices of Western-origin multinational companies, OzNappyfree parents are able to reimagine their minority practice as a global majority practice. In fact, a variety of other global EC-like practices also inform their hygiene assemblage.

Until recently, EC literature has not drawn on Asian practices very explicitly.[16] In popular EC literature, the most commonly cited academic article on "other hygienes" is a 1977 article by deVries and deVries[17] that outlines the basics of EC according to ethnographic work among the Digo people of East Africa. DeVries and deVries argue that in light of Digo toilet training practices, which enable dryness from four to six months, sociocultural factors are more important determinants of toilet training readiness than had been previously thought. They then apply this argument to the United States, showing through a review of historical toilet training advice that sociocultural factors have indeed played a large part in determining readiness.

As part of their argument, deVries and deVries cite a number of reviews of historical literature on toilet training recommendations in three United

States women's magazines between 1890 and 1948, mostly to show how these have changed over the years. (The research they base this on was published in the early 1950s.) Of course, magazine recommendations on toilet training reflect the dominant professional discourses of parenting and toilet training at that time in the United States, not the actual diversity of practices present. But magazine recommendations can reflect popular expectations and ideals. One of the main sociocultural factors affecting toilet training techniques was the increasing emphasis on the soldierly disciplines of routine, obedience, and coercion during the period spanning the world wars. The authors note that the toilet training norms shifted from a mother-centered perspective—where the mother was responsible for ascertaining the right moment to introduce toilet learning—to a practice of rigid scheduling that was based on the assumption that children just needed to be disciplined into toileting. This soldierly toileting discipline includes practices such as tying children to potties until they perform at set times every day and punishments for pottying accidents. This coincides with other changes in caregiving practices at the time, such as strict, routinized feeding and sleeping meant to produce independent and tough future soldiers.[18]

In the United States at least, this was followed by a swing toward more permissive, child-oriented toilet training recommendations in the postwar period. People became more concerned with the psychological effects of coercive toilet training and tended to use rewards and encouragement in conjunction with later toilet training. Although some might read these changes in toilet training techniques teleologically, in that United States women's magazines are reflecting a gradual improvement or evolution in understanding of child behavior and development, deVries and deVries read this as illustrating the sociocultural situatedness of toilet training, given that "infant care writers changed opinions in unison, without the benefit of strong empirical evidence."[19]

DeVries and deVries are careful to distinguish Digo "gentle conditioning" approaches from the "early readiness, rigid environmental scheduling" of the wartime period in the West, preferring to link the Digo approach with the child-oriented approach of their contemporaries in the United States, where infants are imagined as "active participants in training, at quite different times, and prove equally successful."[20] They note that Digo parents also have concepts of the physical and emotional development of infants resulting in a perceived optimal time for bowel and bladder training, yet clearly these are at a different time from those favored by the "matura-tional approach" then (and still) current in the United States. They argue that because "this comparison across cultural settings suggests varied and contradictory possibilities, the maturational explanation for training success should be reevaluated," concluding:

> Expectations and perceptions of infant capabilities and their subsequent translation into behavior are adaptive and attuned to environmental and cultural factors. Concepts of physical maturation are similarly responsive to these factors. Contrary to the current view that all early training is ineffec-tive and/or coercive, maturational timing and "readiness" ideas are related to success only in the way they fit into the total rearing milieu. Readiness is a consequence of a group or family's conceptual and functional ability to carry out a nurturant conditioning technique, and is probably limited only by the individual infant's biologic constraints.[21]

In light of the "multiple infant training possibilities across cultures and over time," they go on to recommend that pediatricians and clinicians take into account the "potential diversity and effect of maternal and fam-ily expectation" and not dogmatically advocate for a "seemingly scientific" approach, especially in medical practices with racially and ethnically het-erogeneous clientele. Forty years down the track, most pediatricians and child health practitioners in Western nations have yet to take up the gaunt-let thrown down by deVries and deVries, even if a growing number of par-ents and urologists have.[22] Some cynics would blame this on the extensive marketing techniques of disposable nappy companies. In recent years, med-ical researchers have begun to explore cultural diversity in infant toileting. One interesting example is the work of Duong, Jansson, and Hellström, published in 2013, documenting the experiences of forty-seven children in Vietnam who were toilet trained over several years. It provides an overview of early toileting patterns and compares them with Swedish infants.[23]

EC in Australia and New Zealand is increasingly well known; it has spread from alternative parenting circles to some mainstream circles in the form of part-time EC. I receive requests from relatively mainstream par-enting groups in both countries to speak on the topic or conduct a work-shop. Despite this wider acceptance in parenting circles, it does seem to be that those who go on to practice EC tend to practice a relatively hands-on attachment parenting[24] or natural parenting[25] baby-care style. These parenting approaches provide a good fit with EC practice because, like caregiving practices in China, they advocate keeping babies close and in arms and being responsive to their nonverbal communications. Most of the more profuse contributors on the OzNappyfree forum are highly educated mothers who understand the implications of attachment research on parenting, but they vary in their adherence to "natural" parenting or attachment parenting ideas and practices. Some, such as Ainslie and Amber, are ardently enthusiastic about all things natural, including being highly suspicious of vaccines or medical interventions. Others, such as Nadine and Janine, are more inclined to practice what works for them socially and culturally, or, in the case of Kerryn and Jen, to use their postgraduate science degrees to access the scientific evidence for a variety of caregiving, hygiene, and health options before choosing.

Rather than viewing EC as only an attachment parenting practice, however, there is recognition within both the Yahoo! Groups and contemporary Facebook groups that various forms of EC are present all over the world and throughout history. A number of OzNappyfree members posted about the positive responses they have received from grandparents and great-grandparents who toilet trained their children early, as well as some members whose parents were from various parts of Asia. Other ECers reported conversations with immigrant mothers at playgroups and other places, delighted that they were "not the only ones" practicing early toileting awareness. While not all these practices completely overlap with EC, there is a definite sense of being a part of a global and historical community of practice, which could even be the majority practice of infant hygiene worldwide.[26]

It was this sense that contributed to the desire of Australian ECers to hear more about my experiences and research in northwest China. During an EC meet-up in Brisbane in 2009, I presented a summary of baniao practice in Qinghai province. This prompted ECers to reflect on the different sociocultural spaces of parenting they inhabited compared to more EC-friendly places. ECers openly disagreed with people who painted a picture of EC as a "third world practice," which only worked because "over there" they "can just do it anywhere" because "babies can only hold on long enough to get to the gutter" (to quote Nadine's father-in-law). They imagined a more idyllic EC lifestyle enabled by a society, such as China, where it was broadly accepted. They thought that the broad acceptance of EC in other societies would relieve the pressure of having to prove EC to be a completely reliable and hygienic method, which results in better and earlier toilet training. They also thought that the living conditions in Xining allowed for more relaxed EC practices (that is, no carpet and a considerable amount of time spent outdoors or in a courtyard) because the basic toilet training rules were "not on the bed or couch" rather than "in the potty or toilet."[27]

Because of the social, spatial, and cultural environment of Australasia, OzNappyfree ECers must work a bit harder to establish EC practices that allow their children to develop toileting awareness without pressuring them. Many ECers try to reduce any pressure on the children to perform in this unsupportive environment by using nappies or training pants as backup, even if their children are pretty reliable. This helps both parent and child better relax in spaces where accidents would not be socially acceptable. Despite these pressures, ECers insist that their children are nevertheless capable of coping with early toileting. Nadine dismisses her skeptical father-in-law's belief that it is not possible in Australia, quipping, "Well, I figured if kids in [other countries] can be toilet trained by 12 months, my kids aren't any more stupid than any of theirs."

Imagining this global community of EC practitioners allows a certain measure of perspective with regards to the cultural specificity of our understandings of hygiene and appropriate toileting behavior, meaning that the child's experience of accidents or misses (a preferred term by many ECers because it emphasizes that the fault is the parent's, not the child's) is rarely negative or disturbing. Imagining a global community of EC is also a strategy that resists the teleological positioning of infant toileting as a backward (and thus dirty and uninformed) care practice. In fact, ECers imagine themselves and the global community of ECers as somewhat progressive, in that science is only just now beginning to catch up with the possibilities of EC. Through imagining the developed world as one which has lost its way in terms of environment and society, and themselves as experimenters drawing on practices in non-Western cultures and places to cultivate alternatives to the overuse of nappies, ECers reposition themselves as being at the forefront of efforts to make a better world. Ainslie, an OzNappyfree mother of two, wonders whether ECers are "the beginning" of a swing away from disposable nappies and late toilet training:

> Perhaps people are starting to see the madness of our disposable nappy driven, 4-year-olds-in-nappies society and we're the beginning of a move back towards early [toilet training] as the norm. (web post, December 2008)

James, a New Zealand father of two, positions the mothers on OzNappy-free as being at the forefront of knowledge around toileting, communicating to the group via his partner, who quoted him as saying:

> You have learnt so much that now you have a trained professional coming to YOU for advice and information. If you had not gained that knowledge and confidence, you have now you would not be able to pass on that information and enrich your community. Be greatful [sic] for what you've got, because it's F***ing BRILLIANT! (in response to a 2009 web post, "Nurse wants to know about EC")

HYGIENE FOR A BETTER WORLD

This chapter has begun to make visible the hygiene and care assemblages gathered around Australian and New Zealand families practicing EC. I have focused on the day-to-day practices of how EC works, linked with an analysis showing how this hygiene assemblage draws on a particular imagining of other hygienes and other places that allows ECers to sidestep teleological ideas of hygienic modernity and development in their caregiving practices.

This builds on the argument made in chapter 1: that it is important to show the bidirectionality of traveling universals and practices between remote areas of China to other parts of the globe. I argue this because I want to both challenge typical analytical frameworks that replay the tired "inevitable emergence of a global era" and steer clear of the equally problematic "culturally relative scraps of data" interpretation of practices and beliefs in out-of-the-way places and spaces.[28] I argue that so-called developed centers of the world need to be open to the fact that there are knowledges and practices in more out-of-the-way places that have relevance for more global contexts, and if we were to look closely, it would be relatively easy to see that these are already traveling.

The fact that relatively educated women in apparent strongholds of hygienic modernity are taking the hygiene knowledges and caregiving practices of women in more out-of-the-way places has serious potential for strengthening the resistance of baniao and similar practices against discourses that position disposable nappy use as more modern and hygienic. The continual coproduction of hygiene assemblages via long distance and awkward, unstable, and even bizarre cross-cultural interactions such as these offers hope that global hygiene homogenization or Westernization is not the only future open to the world. It also shows that changes in these hygiene assemblages can be brought about deliberately. We can tweak and reassemble these hygiene assemblages to better suit the needs of this climate-changing world. The next chapter moves on to explore this reassembling in more detail, where hygiene becomes less about keeping things sparkly clean and more about guarding life and health for our infants and the planet they live on. It is here that some of the radical possibilities of everyday hygiene and care work in embodying a different mode of humanity emerge with more clarity.

Interlude

Experiments

April 2009. Xining, China. I call up my friend, Xiao Shi, and invite her over for lunch. A migrant nanny and domestic worker, Xiao Shi had previously regaled me with stories of rural life and mothering, although by that time her son was a teenager. As we spoke on the phone, she (almost in passing) adds that she "had also given birth." It takes me several seconds to process what she had just said.

"Did you say you have given birth to a child?" I ask in shock. Xiao Shi is Han Chinese, and with a teenage son back in her home province, at that point in time, she is not legally entitled to more children.

"*Shi de,*" she replies. "It is so." She laughs at my shock. "I'm almost forty years old!" she continues, rounding her age up by a good few years. "A little girl, called Yingying. She's four months old."

"Well, you have to bring her over!" I exclaim.

She comes over the following day, and we greet each other with the ease of old friends. She carries baby Yingying in a front pack, huffing up the stairs to our borrowed apartment. She hands over a bag of fruit from her husband's fresh produce shop and shows off a chubby, cheerful baby dressed in many layers of brightly colored and patterned baby clothes.

After lunch, Xiao Shi launches into Yingying's remarkable story, where presumed infertility, long-distance marriage, and an unexpected reunion collaborated to produce an unexpected pregnancy. Despite not being eligible for having a second child under the one-child policy of the time, she decided to go ahead with the birth, which she explains was a result of her Christian faith in God's provision. However, soon after the baby was born, she found she had to give up her main sources of paid domestic work because the

125

family she had previously worked for had also had a second child. The presence of two babies in the house was "too noisy" and "too troublesome," according to Xiao Shi.

"And what of Yingying's household registration?" I ask, knowing that a fine would have to be paid before she could be registered. The fine was more than two years of Xiao Shi's previous full-time earnings, most of which was eaten up week by week. She could no longer work full time, but neither could she go home and face questions from the local authorities. Remaining in Qinghai was a pretty good strategy—except it cut her off from her extended family support networks until the fine could be paid. This pushed a change in parenting style.

This second time around, Xiao Shi's role was less clear than it had been thirteen years earlier in the countryside. In previous conversations in 2007, she had confidently described her role and the role of her mother-in-law, her father-in-law, and her husband with relative clarity. In her village, she was mostly expected to stay close to her child around the home for the first three years, then hand over day-to-day care to her mother-in-law and return to work in the fields. With her son, there was always someone around to hold him, and he slept close to her, feeding as needed throughout the night. When her son started school, she finally weaned him and moved to Xining to seek paid work, as was expected of her. Her income paid for household expenses related to her son back home.

Life is complex, and as Xiao Shi's story illustrates, it can take unexpected turns. She now found herself with a small baby who needed frequent feeding, a husband with a produce shop that barely broke even, and school fees and support owed to her in-laws back home—a home that took more than twenty-four hours to reach by train. She was bound in close proximity to her baby for the time being, but this reduced her availability for paid work, thus compounding her difficulties, even as she insisted on her daughter's right to remain physically close to her for the first two to three years of life.

Perhaps in response to this, Xiao Shi had developed an avid interest in Western parenting practices (after years of disapproval). She had been given a book by a foreigner that advocated for a cry-it-out method of sleep-training babies and provided a parent-directed schedule of feeding and sleeping. Xiao Shi showed me the book when I visited the small concrete produce shop she rented and lived in with her husband and baby. She pulled it out surreptitiously from under her pillow. It turned out to be a translated copy of the controversial baby-training manual *On Becoming Babywise* by American authors Ezzo and Bucknam.

It was an oddly disconcerting juxtaposition of spaces. Xiao Shi and her elderly neighbor discussed the book's contents in a windowless storage room not much wider than the set of iron bunk beds the family retired to nightly. Yet for me, the book's contents conjured an image of a large American-style multistory suburban house, with a separate nursery littered with the paraphernalia of baby care.

Where would you put a baby bed in here? I wondered, noting the simple storage system Xiao Shi and her husband used for their belongings: tying clothing and objects in plastic bags and shoving them in gaps between the bunk beds and the wall, under the bed, and in alcoves in the darkened room. How could you leave a baby to sleep alone in here? You couldn't leave the baby alone on the bunk bed to put herself to sleep; even at four months, Yingying could roll onto the floor in a fit of crying. I wondered who the foreigner was who had gifted this book to Xiao Shi; clearly they had never visited Xiao Shi at home.

The trajectories of this controversial book and that of Xiao Shi's migrant family crossed for a brief moment, providing a flash of insight into the spatiality of different modes of child raising and ways of mothering. She had no mother-in-law present to take on the traditional role of raising Yingying as she returned to work. Like the isolated suburban mother imagined by the *Babywise* authors, Xiao Shi had now found herself in a situation where reducing the demands of her child (rather than merely finding relief from them) was extremely attractive.

The promise held out by *Babywise* fascinated Xiao Shi. It painted a picture of a world of simple order, one in which babies were predictable and mothers were rested and independent. But the book hid under her pillow as if it were contraband or somehow dangerous to her mothering ideals, providing ideas impossible to implement yet attractive. As we spent time discussing the book's contents, Xiao Shi's own nonnegotiables of mothering and child raising came to the fore. Horror and fascination awkwardly engaged as Xiao Shi read *Babywise*, but the engagement allowed her to experiment with different ways of achieving some of its fascinating promises of independence without the horror of neglect.

Xiao Shi experimented with a number of strategies for managing without support. Although she believed the *Babywise* methods to be cruel, she was nevertheless inspired to experiment with less cruel methods. First, she began putting Yingying down for her naps rather than holding her, as was traditional. She gently rocked and fed her until she slept, but then laid her gently on the bed. Through experimentation, Xiao Shi discovered it was not so much that babies needed to be in constant physical contact but that babies needed to be comforted physically if tired or upset and crying.

We discussed this and other experiments we had both conducted in the cross-cultural spaces between us. When I had first begun fieldwork in 2007, Xiao Shi had arrived at my door to ask for work as a cleaner; she had cleaned the house for the previous foreign tenant. I never employed her as a nanny, but her experience in looking after both Chinese and foreign children was the topic of many conversations, and she always took time to greet and speak to my toddler. Xiao Shi had guided me in many experiments as we adapted our hygiene and infant toileting to Xining. She explained how to teach toddlers to squat and urinate on the floor, and how easy it was to mop up afterward. Then, when caregivers see toddlers who needed to go, the caregiver would encourage them to squat (to keep the split-crotch pants from getting wet) and just let it go. Later, you could teach them to go to the bathroom to do it, and eventually the toilet.

I just couldn't. It seemed wrong to encourage her to urinate on the floor. Accidents—yes, fine, there were many. But my response to signs of impending elimination remained intense: swoop in, whisk the child to the bathroom, hold out over the toilet or sink to finish the job. Of course, the intensity of swooping in sometimes inspired resistance, and my hybrid practice remained unskilled despite all the cultural support to do it Xining style. At that point, it wasn't that I believed using the floor to be unhygienic or bad; it was just an embodied, affective response to the concept of urinating on the floor, no doubt habituated into my body when I was around the same age as my child.

Both Xiao Shi and I experimented with parenting on the edge of cultures, sometimes pushed to do so because of new situations. With openness to other ways of doing things, our own practices shifted. Yet they only shifted so far, in line with our embodied knowledge of what just felt right.

5   Reassembling Hygienes

> If to change ourselves is to change our worlds, and the
> relation is reciprocal, the project of making history is never
> a distant one but always right here on the borders of our
> sensing, thinking, feeling, moving bodies.
>
> —J. K. Gibson-Graham, *A Postcapitalist Politics*

> What role can social research play in coming to terms with a
> future in which the certainties of the past have gone and the
> future lies before us unknown? . . . Perhaps we might work
> with lay researchers to help sharpen and strengthen what they
> are doing by applying our critical aptitude in a generous and
> creative spirit.
>
> —Jenny Cameron, "On Experimentation"

Thus far we have mapped out a small part of the hygiene assemblage gathered around the practice of EC as represented by the members of OzNappyfree. This includes the everyday practices of infant toileting for families in
Australia and New Zealand, shaped by the different socialities, spatialities,
and materialities of their particular circumstances. However, as with the
hygiene assemblage in Xining, present-day practices in place are shaped by
a range of converging historical trajectories. In this chapter, I want to map
out the directions of the changes, focusing on the ways their trajectories
converge and reshape the assemblage as they shift and move in relation to
contemporaneous matters of concern. As with the early republican period
in China, many parts of the world are in times of transitional turmoil as
we seek to adapt to a radically altered global situation, both in terms of the
Covid-19 pandemic and adaptation to climate change. At first glance, EC
practitioners might seem to only share an interest in early toilet training,

but there is more here worth investigating: the collective capacity to change both knowledge and habits around an intimate bodily function that has widespread environmental impacts.

In this chapter, I explore the assemblage that is shifting and changing around the practice of elimination communication. EC is, in the Western places I investigate, a shadow hygiene, much like Nie Yuntai's reimagination of a Chinese-style hygiene in the republican era discussed in chapter 3. It represents a new sort of gathering, one that builds on historical trajectories converging in place but also on emerging traveling practices and experimental hybrids. It does not have the power of the state behind it, and it does not have a well-known alternative understanding of the body to draw on, as might be the case with two medical systems operating in one place. What it does have is a group of relatively serious practitioners who are intent on bringing notice to the practice in each cohort of new parents. The current cohort of parents are building their EC knowledges through platforms such as Facebook, TikTok, and Instagram. Many of the same dynamics at play here are the same as those in the parenting groups of the early 2000s from which this research draws: a group of enthusiastic parents who get together to discuss the details of practicing infant toileting. Each person must learn the whole process anew, but each collective of practitioners produces new knowledge built on their experiences and their wider reading and research.

How are these new knowledges built, and what is the relevance to our overall aim of articulating a postdevelopment politics of hygiene? The question of knowledge production is at the heart of the postdevelopment critique as well as the direction of knowledge dissemination. In the case of EC, we have a group of practitioners in Western settings who have limited experience, cultural support, and social knowledge of this hygiene practice. However, rather than assuming that the hygiene knowledges and practices of the Western world are superior, they have placed themselves in the position of learners. This on its own is not enough to be a postdevelopment politics of hygiene, but we can begin to trace the reassembled hygiene as one showing us how change might happen in areas beyond infant toileting.

In what follows, I widen my analysis beyond the practices I observed in my fieldwork. As in chapter 3, I trace other trajectories that are important to the practices on the ground, but in this chapter, I also trace trajectories of possibility—speculative trajectories as much as historical ones. This is not to imply that my analysis of China and hygiene are somehow in the past and static, as opposed to the active and present dynamism that I focus on in this chapter. Rather, this is an appropriate stance to take to think about and analyze a cultural context in which I am an active performer. I see this as similar to what historian Sean Hsiang-lin Lei does in his tracing of a shadow trajectory of hygiene in China's republican era—a cultural context important to him as a Taiwanese academic, and one that, as a historian, he participates in shaping. As J. K. Gibson-Graham remark in the epigraph to this chapter, "The project of making history is never a distant one but always right here on the borders of our sensing, thinking, feeling, moving bodies."[1] The history that we are all part of making together, right now, is the subject of this chapter. Here I weave together trajectories that are part of a reassembled hygiene—a new, more intentional throwntogetherness in the place in which we find ourselves.

History is sometimes envisioned as powerful trajectories of the past that sweep through a place, catching all of us up in forces beyond our control. But it can also be the small and everyday actions that collectively become something powerful enough to cause a swerve in the direction of a trajectory or in the assembling and reassembling of trajectories in place.[2] I return to Val Plumwood's call for "reworking ourselves" and "our high energy, high-consumption, and hyper-instrumental societies."[3] At the beginning of this book, I asked how the deeply embedded and embodied habits of hygiene could be reworked. The changes in China in the first half of the twentieth century give us some sense of how change might happen. Yes, certainly such changes may occur through powerful forces of state and colonialism—but also through the experimental uptake and reworking of practices of the body to fit the moral community, as with Nie Yuntai's shadow trajectory of simple hygiene for all. This can also be seen in the reassembling of individual traditional healers into a collective, primarily in response to the proposal to ban this ancient medical tradition. Members of this group then participated in a politics of collective action at critical moments in deciding on the medical system of the People's Republic. Such a politics of hygiene involves a reworking of the body and society. I have organized the chapter along those two lines, first by detailing the ways in which the bodies of infants and care-givers are affected and reworked through the practice of EC and the awkward engagements that precede it, then by tracing the collective action of hybrid collectives of caregivers, babies, technologies, and practices, all of which share in an embodied reworking of ourselves and our society—or, at the very least, in the reworking and reassembling of hygiene.

AWKWARD BODIES

Awkward engagements between traveling universals are visible in both China and Australia, in a similar way to the global frictions between Indonesia, Japan, and Canada affecting the Kalimantan rain forest Anna Tsing was researching when she coined the term.[4] In the interlude preceding this chapter, I reflected a little bit on the awkward engagement between the infant sleeping norms for American families who followed a strict routine and those such as Xiao Shi, who are accustomed to holding infants while they slept. What is awkward here is also productive. When cultures or practices slip past each other without engaging, we tend to relegate practices as particular to places or spaces that are not our own. What is powerful about awkward engagement between cultures and places, such as Xiao Shi and myself, is the opportunity to think again about our practices, even to rework them. A second awkward engagement occurred when I went to a group meet-up in Birrarung Marr Park in Melbourne.

I attended this meet-up in March 2009. It had been organized via email in a thread for the Melbourne-based EC practitioners on OzNappyfree. I emailed the group and asked if I could come meet them and discuss and observe their EC experiences firsthand. Like the Brisbane group, this group was keen to hear about my research in China. I prepared a few photo collages, printing them out and inserting them in plastic sleeves to hand around. These photos ended up being an eye-opener—not necessarily for the group of mothers who came along, but for myself as I experienced an awkward juxtaposition between the baniao norms demonstrated in the images and the EC practices of those in attendance.

I sat on a concrete step near the playground and introduced myself. I handed around the prepared images. We discussed various differences in the space of practice and community of practice that one might experience in Qinghai in both urban and rural settings. One of the first pictures was of a grandmother and her granddaughter relaxing outdoors in the apartment complex we lived in on Bayi road. As it circulated, Janine, who was sitting next to me on the concrete step, removed her daughter's nappy and sat her on a little portable potty. In a flash, as I became aware of the juxtaposition of those two different images of public spaces and infant toileting, I recognized for the first time the different spatialities of hygiene practice in Xining and Melbourne. Figure 7 shows the image I was showing to the group, along with an image of some mothers sitting on the concrete steps during the meet-up. I wonder how you, the reader, respond to these images?

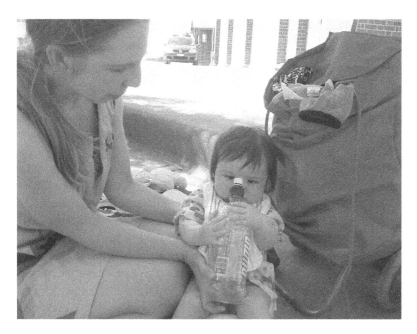

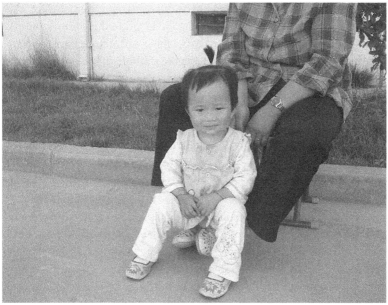

FIGURE 7. An awkward engagement between two hygiene assemblages.
Photographs by author, 2009.

The reader accustomed to hygiene norms in Western countries might view the split-crotch pants of the toddler with bemusement or aversion, but a reader accustomed to hygiene norms in China and other parts of the world might regard people sitting on the ground with similar affective responses. Viewing these two images together clearly shows the different hygiene assemblages. One assemblage gathers objects and practices to keep spaces clean and dry, and one assemblage gathers objects and practices to keep babies' bottoms clean and dry. For me, this particular awkward engagement gave me a chance to connect with a visceral, affect-laden response to different embodied and habituated hygiene universals. My recent time in China collided with the images such that I simultaneously experienced disgust and acceptance for both split-crotch pants (and the implied use of the ground to urinate) and the containment of babies' waste in nappies.

In the two images in Figure 7, the hygiene assemblages of two different spaces are illustrated clearly. In the top image, apart from the unusual sight of a small baby using a potty in a public place, we have a perfect illustration of the norms of hygiene practice in Australia. Janine sits on the ground, as do we all. The baby is seated on a potty, but her bare feet touch the ground. Janine's bag, behind her, is full of the requirements for a day out with a baby. A drink bottle is sitting on the ground too. Once the baby has completed the business in the potty, Janine will remove the little plastic bag in the portable potty and place it in the rubbish. If you were to replace the portable potty with a disposable nappy, you would pretty much have a standard picture of Australian infant toilet hygiene—an assemblage that gathers a variety of materialities and practices to protect the ground from contamination with infant feces or urine.

Keeping hygiene in this community in Australia means protecting oneself and others from contamination by potentially harmful germs. The technique of containment is used to do this, where the potentially harmful germs present in human feces are contained in a potty, toilet, or nappy. Any contamination that results from uncontained eliminations (of any kind—not just disease-carrying feces but also more harmless urine) must be decontaminated by handwashing, floor scrubbing, nappy or clothes washing, and so on. This hygiene assemblage enables (or is enabled by) an intimate bodily engagement with the ground, as illustrated by Janine and her baby. Adults and children may sit, touch, or even lie on the floor or ground in public spaces or homes, with little concern for contamination by disease-carrying matter.[5]

The hygiene assemblage thus includes the materialities of feces and urine and microbes, along with the various receptacles in which they are contained: potties, nappies, toilets, plastic bags. The assemblage also includes the spatialities of engagement with these materialities: floors and ground primarily, but also landfills, sewerage systems and oceans, tree and cotton plantations providing pulp for disposable products, the places and spaces of design and production of products, and even oil extraction for transport or plastic manufacture. The assemblage includes the subjectivities of the children and adults involved—their culturally situated understanding of the body and selfhood developed through their habits of eliminating, decontaminating, and otherwise engaging with spaces, substances, and others. The hygiene assemblage also includes the socialities established through the habituation and normalization of this particular form of hygiene keeping, meaning that challenging this assemblage is not a simple matter of individual decision. Each of these elements is not passively situated in a timeless space but is the result of the dynamics of a variety of historical trajectories, some of which were discussed in chapter 3.

Now consider the bottom image of Figure 7, where a grandmother sits outdoors on a small folding stool on the concrete public area of the apartment complex. Her granddaughter wears split-crotch pants and little shoes and is seated on her grandmother's feet. For both, only the feet are touching the ground. Despite hanging out in the courtyard for most of the day, neither has brought any other possessions along, aside from the stool. There is nothing particularly interesting about this picture for the average Xining resident. It illustrates the hygiene and caregiving assemblage common to Xining, including the practices and relationships that keep hygiene and health. In this picture and in my fieldwork, hygiene is kept in a more overtly spatial and relational way than it is in Australia and New Zealand, using the techniques of imagination and separation. Particular spaces can be imagined as quite dirty, whether visibly so or not, and people might use bodily and relational techniques to separate themselves from the dirty spaces. As is illustrated in this picture, only the feet touch the floor or ground in most situations,[6] and even in newer, tiled houses where the shoes are removed, slippers are worn on the tiled floors.

The ground is generally considered dirty; it is often considerably more dusty and visibly dirty than outdoor spaces in Australia, presumably the result of different, finer soil composition, but also because of coal-fired boilers and car exhaust in the city. Babies and toddlers wear split-crotch pants that enable them to squat and freely urinate in public spaces and some homes. Children are not normally permitted to touch or sit on the ground, even in relatively clean spaces. They are often physically redirected into a squat unless they are seated on a bed, couch, or rug. They are thus consistently habituated into a particular engagement with space, one that requires a strict practice of bodily boundaries between clean and dirty spaces.

When a baby or toddler urinates on the floor, it is cleaned up using a rag-head mop. In rural homes with dirt floors, ashes from the fire are often thrown over urine puddles or feces, and these are swept up and discarded. This continues until a child has learned to walk to the appropriate place and navigate into position over a bathroom drain, squat toilet, or potty.[7] Eventually the child is able to wear ordinary pants and pull them down to use any type of toilet, be it public, Western style, outhouse, or squat. But even after complete toilet independence has been achieved for the young of the household, the ground is still imagined to be essentially a dirty space. It seems that this dirtiness is not necessarily related to the potential trace presence of urine (or even feces); rather, imagining the ground and floor as essentially dirty enables a practice of hygiene that includes allowing infant urine (and sometimes feces) on the floor.

The matter-of-fact acceptance of elimination-related bodily functions is also likely enabled by and enables baniao hygiene. For many centuries in China, "honeypot" collectors gathered and even purchased night waste for use as fertilizer. Excrement thus has a long history of being considered "less a public health matter" and more "an integral element of agricultural production and a precious commodity."[8] Although no longer collected in this way, it is still not uncommon to use human manure for farming in rural China. This is a quite different historical trajectory than what is seen in other parts of the world, where human waste may be considered disgusting, taboo, or spiritually polluting. In this context, in China, the poo and pee of babies is considered a natural part of life.

The hygiene assemblage thus gathered in Xining (as loosely represented in Figure 7) includes these historical trajectories of imagining feces primarily as a resource. It also includes the spatialities of traditional and contemporary housing, waste management, public bathrooms, and farming. It gathers the materialities of dirt, urine, soil, feces, fertilizer, crops, split-crotch pants, potties, mops, cesspits, ashes, concrete, tiles, toilets, and drains. Finally, it includes the different situated subjectivities thus habituated in children and babies and caregivers, played out through different bodily engagements with space and stuff and each other.

The two hygiene assemblages I am concerned with here become more visible when brought into conversation, even if this awkward engagement is primarily a moment of photographic juxtaposition. The moment of awkward engagement illustrated in Figure 7 allows us not only to see hygiene assemblages but also to begin thinking about how they shift, change, and reassemble. It also made visible the emerging assemblage of an Australian version of baniao, where cultural norms of keeping spaces clean and dry could be performed while simultaneously keeping babies' bottoms clean and dry. Like the lazy Susan or hygienic table (and associated practices) that Nie Yuntai and friends used to balance Western and Chinese forms of hygiene, new objects and practices emerge from awkward engagements between universals in what Anna Tsing calls friction, because it is in the sparking and gripping of these awkward engagements that movement and change might happen.[9] But a spark and some friction do not necessarily produce change—and when they do, what exactly is happening? I have found the language of "learning to be affected" helpful in thinking this through.[10]

LEARNING TO BE AFFECTED

The awkward engagement discussed above, as well as the ones in the interlude preceding this chapter, shed light on some sort of difference in practice and include an engagement with difference. Such an engagement with difference may increase possibilities for doing things differently. Bruno Latour has spent some time thinking about how this change might happen, particularly when it comes to the body. He uses the language of "learning to be affected" to describe the ways in which a body comes to "interface" with its surroundings in such a way as to increase its capacity act.[11] To recast this notion in terms of my argument here, learning to be affected is something that can happen through an awkward engagement, where conflicting or curious trajectories clash or engage in some way that (in the body) seems awkward. However, this does not have to apply to all cases.

Latour uses the example of the Nose, a person trained in the perfume industry through the use of odor kits until able to distinguish a wide range of odors not distinguishable to those who have not learned to be affected in this way.[12] Jenny Cameron and colleagues use the idea to think about how people can learn to be affected by country, by climate, by butterflies and bees, and by gardens in a way that is embodied and not easily rationalized.[13] Neither of these necessarily requires an awkward engagement; nor does EC. While people might come to learn about EC or baniao through an awkward engagement, such as unexpectedly seeing an infant being held out, in contexts where the practice is normalized, it is more about intentionally cultivating a new sense. Both EC and baniao practices rely on such a period of learning to be affected, where caregivers deliberately tune themselves into the subtle signs and signals of impending elimination. As these become increasingly differentiated, the baby also learns to be affected by the particular responses and cues of their caregivers, increasing their ability to communicate and thus act in response.

In Xining, this interfacing happens primarily during the *yuezi* lying-in period. During the initial part of this period of thirty to one hundred days, the grandmother or other older caregiver takes responsibility for the baby's eliminations with the support of soft *niaobu* cloths, split-crotch pants, and a wide basin. During this time, the new mother and baby are not permitted to go outside, and in many cases, the mother is also discouraged from watching television, reading, or any other activity. She is encouraged to eat and sleep and make breast milk (through special foods and extra meals). This period is justified mostly in terms of the mother's health, but its adherence also allows a sustained period of learning to be affected by the baby, in particular its signals and patterns for feeding, sleeping, and eliminating. This *yuezi* period is effectively a time of important transitions, where mother, baby, grandmother, and other family members transition into their new relationships and family roles. By the end of the confinement period, the baby's elimination patterns are well known to the family, and the baby responds bodily to holding out and other cues regarding elimination.

ECers also put themselves through a period of training and learning to be affected. Some begin by removing their baby's nappy and holding it wrapped in a towel for a certain amount of time each day, making an effort to observe when the baby eliminates and any signs that precede this. Others may take note of the common signs listed by others on OzNappyfree or in books on the subject. When their babies appear to give one of these signs, they respond by holding the baby in position over a potty, bucket, or sink. The process of response is an important part of learning to be affected. With this relationship, if signs are not responded to, then the conversation is one-sided and eventually grinds to a halt. If the signs are responded to promptly and consistently over time, they may develop into more deliberate signals through reinforcement and response. Eventually the ECing caregiver may also develop an embodied intuition that does not require deliberate signals and responses because they have learned to be bodily affected by the baby's signs.

In both Chinese and Australian baniao/EC practices, the bodies of caregiver and baby are each affected or moved by such interfacing. While some caregivers rely more on timing and keeping track, for most, the practice becomes intuitive over time. Bodies entangle and (re)connect, forming a caregiver–baby collective that is more differentiated than the mother–baby collective embodied in pregnancy. The human, the more than human, and even the intrahuman interact in concert and disconsonance. Hormones, microbes, gases, and chimeric cells shared between birth mother and child all trouble our notions of intentionality and agency. But a whole-body learning to be affected has increased this caregiver–baby collective's options for hygiene-keeping action.

The increased capacity to act through an increasingly differentiated world is the point here; learning to be affected is the way this happens. The increased capacity to act is perhaps initially at a more individual or household level, and this may be understood by some to be another example of the problematic way that collective concerns, such as hygiene, health, and environmental action, come to be responsibilized to nuclear families. However, let us not be too hasty in lining this up with that pattern. As Gerda Roelvink reminds us, when we learn a constellation (such as neoliberalism), we tend to see that arrangement of stars first whenever we look at the sky rather than the billions of other possible combinations and patterns of affect and effect.[14] The increased capacity to act for different forms of hygiene widens possibilities; indeed, it widens possibilities for new kinds of collectives.

The capacity to respond to differentiated signals allows a shift in the mode of care; rather than a more powerful individual caring about or caring for an infant's hygiene, it shifts us to a more collaborative mode of caring *with*. For care theorist Joan Tronto, this greater capacity to "care with" is of political importance. It enables us to move beyond *homo economicus,* a "rational economic man," to *homines curans,* a "collective caring subject," where people can "rely on an ongoing cycle of care to continue to meet their caring needs."[15] In what follows, I examine the more collective aspects of this reassembled infant hygiene, in which EC caregivers and families form part of a hybrid care collective with increased collective capacity to act.

COLLECTIVE KNOWLEDGE MAKING

We began back in chapter 1 by acknowledging the multiplicity of worlds and trajectories and bodies and realities to be part of a postdevelopment and postcolonial project. In acknowledging such multiplicity, we must also acknowledge how far these multiplicities interact and coassemble. We have seen how different forms of hygiene exist around the world, and how these worlds of hygiene interact through traveling practices—and indeed universals. We have seen how entire empires of hygiene are made and remade through interactions of multiple historical trajectories in place. We have seen how our ghosts or our shadow hygienes (and realities) have quietly reproduced in the shadow of nation-states, power plays, and medical universals of the body. We have seen how practices of hygiene, such as EC, have sprouted and flourished and shifted hygienes in diverse places, and we have thought a little bit about how this happens through the awkward engagements of universals and through the process of learning to be affected by new embodied realities that multiply possibilities and therefore increase our capacity to act, even across and between different hygiene realities. At this point of the book, however, I want to turn to our larger collective problems of hygiene and pull together these different ideas to say something about how intentional change might proliferate, both in the area of hygiene but also more broadly.

One of the things I have struggled with as I have dived into the EC world are the critiques in the back of my mind—the ones that sneak up and whisper quietly, "But isn't this all neoliberal individualization of what should be public responsibility?" I think of work by Kate Cairns, Norah MacKendrick, and Josée Johnston, where they found mothers of many different class and race backgrounds felt pressure to individually research, source, and prepare organic food for the sake of their child's health (as well as the environment). Some, of course, were unable to do so, and feelings of guilt ensued.[16] They argue that the burden of changing the food system should not be placed on the shoulders of mothers alone. They are right, of course, but what should we say of the work that mothers do in the areas of environment and parenting, and how do we collectivize such work in the way that Cairns and colleagues recommend? In the case of EC, this means asking what happens once a mother (mothers in particular, but also others) has learned to be affected by an issue of environmental or social importance, and how do we move beyond personal responsibility alone in addressing it?

In my other research work, I have found that change often begins with small groups of people who assume responsibility to do things differently—not necessarily in the hope of completely changing a system but to work out some of the finer details on how to live differently in place. In the years following the devastating earthquakes in Christchurch, New Zealand, for example, we found that individuals and small groups began some of the transformative and transitional work of recovery by experimenting in vacant lots.[17] A kitsch garden and a pavilion made of pallets for wind protection in community events were some of the early projects of Gap Filler. The public response to these interventions, at a time when 80 percent of the central city was slated for demolition, fed into the creation of a number of charitable trusts. Some put together interventions for shared wellbeing in the city, and one acted as a matchmaker between landowners of vacant lots and the artists, entrepreneurs, educators, and creatives who might activate them. Ten years later, three of these organizations are supported by the city council with responsibilities for ongoing place-making and urban development, and they even contribute to such work in other regional and suburban areas.[18] What began as small-scale experiments, where individuals and small groups took responsibility for initiating small changes, became partially publicly funded with shared responsibility for caring for a variety of common spaces in the city, including privately and publicly owned lands.

For those involved in OzNappyfree, people have taken responsibility for learning new ways of doing hygiene, often individually. However, the collectivization of the work becomes apparent through the shared work of the forum. The forum at the time of my research was not merely a discourse that influenced parents but a shared experimental endeavor. Any sense of personal responsibility that arose from it is not necessarily in the same vein as the mother-blaming discourses that Cairns and colleagues note around food and nutrition. The forum was a space where mothers (and one father) reflected on their parenting practices and explored the limits of their care labor alongside other possibilities. Thematic analysis of the OzNappyfree posts of 2009 revealed themes of sustainable consumption and infant attachment (areas that require increased responsibility and labor for mothers seeking to ensure these outcomes), but also strong themes

of balancing caring labor with other needs and collectively caring for an
EC knowledge commons.[19] Many referred to themselves as lazy parents
who could not be bothered with nappies, routine, or extra baby equipment.
Melanie, for example, posted:

> Some people think of EC as a lot of hard work—but I'd much rather flush a
> toilet than clean a bottom. . . . There's also the thrill of the catch—my partner
> and I still get a kick out of it and discuss the results. (web post, January 2008)

Mothers counseled one other to take care, and those who lived close
enough also met and provided tangible support. While some reported feeling anxious and perfectionist about their EC practice, the forum was not a
perfectionist space; failures were reported as often as success.[20] As such,
although there is some evidence for responsibilization, it is no more or less
than the everyday responsibilization of care that parents have experienced
for generations. Indeed, the forum was a space where collectives might
begin to loosely form.

These loose collectives were the beginning of small change, in much
the same way that loose collectives of place-making creatives began the
transformative work in Christchurch. With many details still left to iron
out, and few definitive sources of advice and research, the OzNappyfree
collective approached the practice of EC as an open-ended experiment,
with collective sharing and discussion of findings. This contrasts with cloth
nappy forums and Facebook groups, and indeed even breastfeeding groups,
where the facts are known and recited between mothers in ways that reinforce the social norms of the group.[21] Experiments included regular data
collection in the form of monthly reports on each child—at least when time
allowed. These reports followed a relatively standard format. Like Latour
and Woolgar's study of the laboratory where scientific facts were made,[22]
OzNappyfree included experiments (parents trialing new approaches with
babies), inscriptions (writing up the results and posting them on the forum),
statements (of the findings), disputes (between other experimenters), and
finally, settlement of the facts. Knowledge making within OzNappyfree is
thus something like a lay science, with people testing, experimenting, and
refining what is true in collaboration with others.

It was not only a process of knowledge making that crossed over with
science, however; there was also significant crossover with the processes
Judith Farquhar and Lili Lai summarize as the ways in which different

minority nationality medicines are collectively recovered and formalized in modern-day China.[23] They report that the processes of salvaging, sorting, synthesizing, and elevating are carried out all over the minority regions of the country, uplifting the different medical practices of different cultural groups in much the same way the Han-dominated TCM was developed. In the context of OzNappyfree, salvaging involves finding old knowledges of EC and baniao, as well as documenting practices and experiences. Sorting involves collectively and individually working out what will work in Australian and New Zealand contexts. Synthesizing could refer to bringing together a variety of knowledges and formalizing the coherence between them—often in this case in books, articles, or websites that members have developed, but also research. Elevating refers to sharing of knowledge more widely. Knowledge making on the OzNappyfree forum is thus something akin to gathering a new body practice of health. Perhaps it is even a new ontology within a pluriverse—a knowledge that is, perhaps, more than scientific.

Whatever the framework used, research, experimentation, and knowledge making were being done. Caregivers deliberately experimented with different assemblages of potties, clothing, timing, spaces, and so on, and reported their results. Others read books and articles and interviewed other people (such as older people, and people from cultures where forms of EC were practiced widely), again reporting their results. Caregivers brought questions to the group to be answered—some moral and ethical, some practical, some scientific. People offered their different skills in response: an occupational therapist specializing in children offered advice on phobias, a nutritionist and a nurse offered advice on food allergies and EC, and I shared what I knew of EC/baniao practice in China. The open-ended experiment of the forums has a lot of resonance with the work of Michel Callon and Vololona Rabeharisoa and the hybrid research work of the French association for muscular dystrophy, Association Française contre les Myopathies (AFM).[24] In the next section, I use the AFM's work on hybrid collectives to think about the experimental work carried out by the OzNappyfree hybrid collective in the wild.

HYBRID COLLECTIVES AND RESEARCH IN THE WILD

The experimentation and knowledge production of OzNappyfree is, as discussed above, a form of research. It is not to say that it is the same kind of exacting research conducted by trained researchers and scientists; it is instead a different form of research, one Callon and Rabeharisoa call research in the wild—that is, research outside the formal academy. Callon and Rabeharisoa developed the concept through their work with AFM. The association collaborates with professional scientists to produce useful new knowledge about the disease. In the case of muscular dystrophy, the embodied experience of the disease is critically important for knowledge about the disease, but it is difficult to study from the outside or in the laboratory. Patients and parents thus develop methods to document life with muscular dystrophy for use by scientists. They use photos, journals, testimonies, and so on to collect and convey the diversity of bodily experiences of life with muscular dystrophy. Callon and Rabeharisoa propose that "it might be fruitful to consider concerned groups as (potentially) genuine researchers, capable of working cooperatively with professional scientists. In so doing, they invent a new form of research, which we propose to call research 'in the wild.'"[25]

Gerda Roelvink points out that the organization's research "disrupted the discourse representing patients as . . . a single homogeneous terminal case."[26] In a similar way, OzNappyfree parents (and Xiao Shi and her neighbor, mentioned in the interlude) use methods that capture embodied experiences and connections to produce knowledge that differentiates the variety of babies' bottoms and experiences of sphincter control, toileting, communication, and so on. Such embodied methods might not be possible in formal medical research. The research in the wild also disrupts a medical discourse of homogeneity—in this case, the presumed homogeneity of the infant sphincter and infant communication, and hence toileting capabilities.

Researching embodied experiences is not the only reason for research in the wild, however; sometimes professional researchers are just not as motivated to research matters of deep concern for particular groups in society. More domesticated forms of research have traditionally been organized around matters of fact rather than matters of concern or matters of care. Such research has intended to produce more and more accurate facts about the world and its inhabitants within particular disciplines.[27] Increasingly, social scientists are doing research that does more than just critique or uncover facts, and there is a groundswell of affirmative and reparative forms of critique that work to construct possibilities in particular areas of concern.[28] But for researchers in the wild, organizing around matters of care is a distinctive feature of their work, which is mostly uninhibited by the established disciplines of professional research and motivated by things

that affect them personally and deeply. It has even been argued that historically, it has been amateurs in the wild who have made breakthroughs in
research fields as disparate as computing, paleontology, and physics pre-
cisely because of their ability to obsess over a matter of care and go against
established wisdom.[29]

In the case of OzNappyfree, the collective (and I) argue that contrary to
popular belief in Australia and New Zealand, babies can actively participate in toileting, even when just a few days old. They may not be able to
physically hold in urine for significant periods of time, but they can actively
release their sphincter muscle and thus respond to toileting cues. If babies
continue to practice releasing their sphincter muscle, it is possible for the
exercise to enable full bladder control to develop well before the age of
two years—the age cited as normal in Australia and New Zealand. But how
do OzNappyfree members and ECers (and I) know this? Is this knowledge
reliable? How does their research process compare to that of a university
or medical researcher?

In the case of muscular dystrophy, Callon and Rabeharisoa point out
that research is necessary in both laboratory and wild contexts. They argue
that lay and scientific research are complementary, refusing to place one
over and above the other as the final arbiter of truth or usefulness. The
parent practitioners of EC would no doubt agree; in fact, many of them
work within the medical establishment as nurses, midwives, doctors, and
therapists, and others work in universities as scientists or researchers, or are
studying in any one of these fields. Most of the members actively drew on
scientific research in theorizing and making claims about their EC practice.
Yet in some significant points, the knowledge produced by OzNappyfree
contradicts that of the medical establishment and published research. Sometimes the areas of research interest to OzNappyfree members are of little
interest to the wider research community (or funding bodies). Research
questions such as "how can we care for both infants and planet by keeping
hygiene in a more sustainable way, without hygiene products?" is a question
not likely to be funded in medical research, and certainly not in corporate
product development research. Moving forward in producing knowledge
about EC is therefore done almost entirely through hybrid collectives of
lay researchers.

As Callon and Rabeharisoa narrate the story of muscular dystrophy
research in France, for research with and by AFM, "there is no fundamen-
tal difference of status between knowledge produced by patients and that

produced by researchers or clinicians."[30] Indeed, the partnership between the patients, researchers, and clinicians and the prostheses, genes, animal subjects, technologies, and more permits the formation of a new collective entity that might be called a hybrid collective. However, the hybrid collective is not a circumstantial assemblage, a multiplicity of historical trajectories, or an awkward engagement, as we have examined earlier in this book. It is a deliberately assembled group, one with intention. As Callon and Rabeharisoa put it: "The collaboration that builds up between researchers in the wild and laboratory specialists allows this exploration and joint construction of the hybrid collective."[31] The hybrid collective is an intentional community—in this case, a community caring for the specific knowledge commons of muscular dystrophy treatment and knowledge. Even skeptics looking at what the AFM is doing would say that this is individualizing or outsourcing patient care to nuclear families, although they might argue that more public support should be forthcoming. It is my proposition that the work of OzNappyfree can also be read as a hybrid collective, an intentional community that has come together to care for the knowledge commons of EC and to disseminate this knowledge further afield.

The concept of hybrid collectives has been used by a few different scholars to think about intentional social change in a way that includes the active agency of nonhuman others. J. K. Gibson-Graham and Gerda Roelvink adopt the notion of the hybrid research collective to explain the ways in which their own work has been a process of learning together, with human and more-than-human others. Roelvink describes the way in which she, as a researcher at the World Social Forum, became part of a "hybrid collective creating new worlds" and "enacting a new econo-sociality."[32] Roelvink describes the hybrid collective, which included all the other participants acting together and all that made the forum possible (technologies, tents, food markets, and so on). Jenny Cameron and colleagues use the concept to apply to the kinds of collectives formed between community gardeners in Australia, including the different gardeners and their organizations, as well as the technologies that brought them together, including buses and radio. They have identified the ways in which hybrid collectives gather, reassemble, and translate knowledge in the context of community food economies in the Philippines and Australia.[33] I have written with colleagues about hybrid care collectives, hybrid activist collectives, and hybrid research collectives, which in turn each do the work of care, activism, and research collectively, in a range of different settings.[34]

What I think the concept adds to the idea of more-than-human assemblages is the concept of collective, intentional endeavors. That is, they do something, and for a purpose, whether it is a gathering of knowledges, an experimental research process, or caring for a knowledge commons. Although an assemblage is certainly active and acting, there is less of a sense of intentionality in its actions; its list of trajectories might be amorphous and shifting. The happenstance throwntogetherness of the assemblage is not what a hybrid collective represents.[35] The hybrid collective acts with intentionality and with shared purpose, even if elements might sometimes be contradictory or at cross-purposes. This hybrid collective includes a community of subjects—perhaps giving insight into Tronto's *homines curans,* the collective, caring subject—but in this case insisting that such a subject is more than human.[36] In a community economy, a hybrid collective is also used to identify the commoning community—that is, the community that takes responsibility and cares for a particular commons.[37] Thus, the hybrid collective has an important role to play in intentional change—in this case, in assembling and reassembling hygienes. But what is the process by which such a hybrid collective comes to act collectively for different outcomes, for new worlds? Let us return once again to the concept of learning to be affected.

REASSEMBLING AFFECTIVE HYGIENES

The hybrid research collectives of OzNappyfree are made up of smaller household-level collectives, often composed of mothers and babies, or other caregivers and babies. As detailed earlier, caregivers and babies come to learn to be affected by each other—caregivers by the nonverbal communications and signs used by babies to indicate their need to eliminate, and babies by the positions and cues set up by caregivers to indicate and assist with releasing the sphincter muscles. However, learning to be affected is not only about the embodied interfacing of these small collectives of two or more in an intense caregiving and care-receiving relationship. These smaller collectives are also engaged in a broader collective process of learning to be affected, or "caring with."

Through the practice of EC, OzNappyfree members had already learned to be affected by the unspoken communications of their children, but there was also a wider collective process of learning to be affected. I personally came to experience this after a series of hair-washing battles with my then two-year-old daughter. In desperation, I posted to the off-topic group about my issues with hair washing, asking for suggestions to elicit my daughter's cooperation that would respect her communications of dislike. Instead, I received from group members a (surprising) challenge to my insistence on hair washing, in light of some discussions that had already played out about the unnecessary use of cleaning products such as shampoo.

Another group of parents may have just insisted that children learn to cope with hair washing, but this group had already learned to be deeply affected by their children's nonverbal communications in the practice of EC. Beginning from the assumption that my daughter had a valid reason for her resistance, various members researched and posted links to information on the chemicals in shampoo and toothpaste and the reasons for their inclusion in standard products (they are a cheap way to add foam, which we habitually expect from these products). Others posted links to research articles and radio programs on skin health and dermatology. Others posted their experiments with alternatives such as baking soda and apple cider vinegar, going into excruciating detail about how to make it work. Others posted their long-term reflections on this (one mother of teenage daughters, for example), while others posted in detail the day-to-day progress until their body adjusted to life without shampoo.

Here, it is clear that through an openness to listening to the child other, an entire collective research endeavor was spawned. There was a salvaging, a sorting, a synthesizing, and—eventually—an elevating of the knowledge of hair hygiene. I was not the first or last to ask this question, and as it regularly came up, the process repeated and refined, where statements and disputes were settled, until a number of research conclusions seem to have been collectively reached:

Shampoo is unnecessary for good hygiene, and certain kinds are harmful to
   the health of skin and eyes, as well as waterways.
You can wash your hair with just hot water and a lot of rubbing.
You can do this irregularly with children yet have no smelliness, oiliness, or
   dirtiness, provided you brush or comb out any food or anything else that
   gets in their hair.
Alternatives to shampoo that have been shown to work well (by this collective) are a paste of baking soda and water, followed by a rinse with apple
   cider vinegar and water; conditioner only; Sorbolene; eggs; lemon juice;
   and rosemary-infused water.

It takes a period of time for your hair to adjust to a different regimen, and
this may involve a period of oiliness. Brushing the hair a lot seems to help
redistribute the oil. Eventually the scalp settles down and stops producing so much oil (theorized to be a response to the stripping effects of
shampoo).

Hair may appear to be different color or have a different texture from what
one has become accustomed to under a shampoo regimen.

Cleaning hair has been done differently in different places and in different
historical periods.

Some types of hair do not respond well to this regimen, especially very fine or
blond hair, a large quantity of hair, or the hair of people who sweat a lot.

People have varying attachments to nice-smelling hair, which can be achieved
by using light sprays of water with added essential (or coconut) oil, as is
common in India.

A number of organic, plant-based herbal products such as shampoo bars are
available in Australia and New Zealand that can be used by those who do
not seem to adjust to no 'poo, as the practice is often called. Those not
willing to go completely no 'poo can greatly reduce the frequency of hair
washing with shampoo through a transition period.[38]

The hybrid research collective gathered around OzNappyfree came to
be affected by children's communications of discomfort to such a degree
that the hygiene regimen came to be questioned before the child. Rather
than attempting to habituate or discipline children into hygienic modernity, the group gathered a vast assemblage of information from formal
academic sources and lay experimentation to support a child's communication. This type of experimentation not only sparked new thinking about
hygiene possibilities but also resulted in changes in material conditions and
even in subjectivity. In some ways, the hybrid collective participated in creating a different, shared world of hygiene—a different hygiene reality. In
a concrete way, the hybrid collective was able to tweak the assemblage
toward one that better cares for the needs of babies and ecosystems. Now,
in 2023, shampoo bars and "no 'poo" hair-care regimens are relatively normalized.[39] Other experiments included, of course, the details of EC, but also
the use of menstrual cups and the development of homemade cloth menstrual pads, which are also now relatively normalized; commercial versions
can be bought in supermarkets and pharmacies near my home in New
Zealand, as well as in ninety-eight other nations.[40]

The hybrid collective enacted—and continues to enact—a particular hygiene reality through experiments for socioecological change while prioritizing care and embodied connection with babies and children. The hybrid collective has learned to be affected and has increased its capacity to act by creating a social space where different forms of hygiene are carefully (re)assembled. The new, shared worlds of hygiene have spread beyond the enthusiastic experimenters of OzNappyfree and their environmentalist circles and become part of the ordinary hygiene realities of wider groups as information and equipment for these reassembled hygienes becomes translated and more easily available to those who are not actively seeking alternatives.[41] The increased capacity to act then widens its circle, reaching even those who are not really interested in reassembling hygiene. This is perhaps a sketch of what a postdevelopment politics of hygiene might look like: hybrid collectives working in experimental ways to produce hygiene knowledges adapted to place and with care for both humans and the environment.

GUARDING LIFE IN TIMES OF TRANSITION

Hygiene as defined by the biomedical tradition is but one trajectory that has informed the reassembling of hygienes discussed in this chapter. That tradition, relying heavily as it does on understandings of contamination and decontamination and the prerogative to keep spaces clean and dry, is one that has informed the reassembled hygiene of OzNappyfree. But we are only partway along that trajectory, and other trajectories are converging. In biomedicine, there is an increasing understanding of the role of the microbiome in keeping health, as well as evidence that killing germs and decontamination are not the only, or even best, ways to do hygiene when the microbiome's biodiversity is at stake.[42] As other trajectories interact with this trajectory, there is space for experiments and new knowledge making.

This chapter has detailed how the new knowledge making around hygiene has emerged from processes of learning to be affected by other bodies, which increases individual capacities to act. It has detailed how new knowledge making around hygiene has occurred through hybrid collectives experimenting and researching in the wild, and in turn learning to be affected collectively. The increased collective capacity to act has thus informed the kinds of hygienes that emerge from the experiments of the OzNappyfree group. I have selected just a single example of learning to be affected, but there are many possibilities. For example, learning to be affected by plastic packaging prompted hygiene rethinking in the areas of menstrual products, where one disposable pad can include as many as four plastic bags' worth of plastic. The collective knowledge making around hair washing, reusable menstrual products, and more came alongside the knowledge making surrounding nappy-free infant toileting. Accordingly, if the hybrid collective is the entity making new knowledges, then what happens to these knowledges, and how are they cared for? How are these new hygiene knowledges incorporated into realities? Into different kinds of shared hygiene futures?

Here I return to the language used of hygiene in China: *weisheng,* guarding life. What I propose is that we—you and I, those of us in the privileged space to be reading such books at this time—adopt a notion of hygiene as guarding life. What does it mean to guard life, and how does this play on the word *hygiene* help us move forward into a postdevelopment politics of hygiene? How do we think about change and our hygiene futures—change that builds from the ordinary, everyday realities of families and places trying to live the best life they can in difficult times, rather than the technoindustrial-engineered realities of global sanitation and hygiene consultants? If our starting point is guarding life rather than reproducing Western realities everywhere in the world, what would social change look like? How would we adapt our practices to guard life in all its forms—the oceans, the coasts, the forests, the mountains, the rivers, the wetlands, and all the life that teems (or should be teeming) in them? As we have seen in this chapter, a hybrid collective might gather to make changes by performing experimental work, learning to be affected, and reassembling seemingly solid assemblages in new ways. What might this mean in our challenging times? This is where we proceed next.

6 Guarding Life

In this new Earth era, it seems that we are overdue for a new, different mode of humanity that enables caring ways of living with our planet and with each other. At the beginning of this book, I asked what a different mode of hygiene might look like, and what a researcher such as myself might offer such a project without falling into neocolonial development teleologies that assume that West is best. As part of the unfolding journey of answering that question, I often returned to Gerda Roelvink's words on collective action in a climate-changed world. In her contribution to *Manifesto for Living in the Anthropocene,* she asks researchers to "seek out those who are already transforming their relationships with the more than human world, to learn about and tell their stories, and to help multiply, magnify, legitimate, and proliferate their practice."[1]

This has inspired me to think about how scholars might cultivate regenerative, transformative, postdevelopment thinking for change through more consciously opening ourselves to the multiple contemporaneous realities already present. In what has come before in this book, I have rejected teleological arguments that assume change comes about through global homogenization. Instead, I have worked to seek out, multiply, and magnify diversity through detailed accounts of changes that have come about through complex and contingent interactions between multiple trajectories, multiple modernities, and multiple realities. I have sought out the diverse embodied hygiene realities of those who gather different socialities, spatialities, and materialities into hygiene assemblages, such as those present in contemporary Xining and those meeting virtually on OzNappyfree. Like Roelvink, I have found that indeed there are many who are engaged in learning from our climate-changed Earth in such a way that they themselves are transformed and are prompted to create new ways of living with others.

In this book, I have found particular inspiration from the many mothers and grandmothers working to guard life in their everyday contexts. This guarding life is care work, and, like all care work, it is work that can be deeply transformative. While each caregiving relationship requires both caregiver and care receiver to attenuate to each other, I am interested in Sara Ruddick's claim that the nurturing relationship often embodied by mothers can lead to a particular way of thinking that combines somewhat abstract future goals in the minute decision-making of everyday life.[2] I have seen evidence of this sort of care work in my research here. In the details of how to wash children's hair with no shampoo, exactly how to put a baby to sleep in a way that nurtures both caregiver and infant wellbeing, and the attentive acts of holding out and learning baby's signals for elimination, the caregiver holds in mind the health of the microbiome and planetary waterways, the psychological wellbeing of a future adult and the long journey of parenting to get them there, the end life of disposable products, and the water cycle of their region. The kinds of everyday experimentation of the people I researched in both urban Xining and the OzNappyfree network were the kinds of experimentation required for reassembling hygiene, but also transformation more generally.

I have also shown how hygiene assemblages in contemporary China, Australia, and Aotearoa New Zealand can shift, be reassembled, and provoke change. I have become particularly interested in hybrid human and more-than-human research collectives that do this reassembling work, and the process by which they start to reassemble and provoke change. It seems that the process by which these collectives reassemble hygiene assemblages and provoke change is through the development of different kinds of subjects—adults who are affected and moved by caring for babies and children, and babies and children and adults who are affected and moved by the world around them. This assembling and reassembling is not driven by top-down changes in law or policy but rather emerges from groups of people gathering around matters of shared care and concern.

Yet this is not to say that law and policy are not important for spreading and embedding the experiments of hybrid collectives. This we have seen in the case of China's changing hygiene assemblages in chapter 3, in the world's responses to the Covid-19 pandemic, and in the many shifts that have occurred in recent years spurred by local and national governments.

While many people I know had been using reusable bags at the supermarket for some time, the ban on disposable plastic bags first in China and then in New Zealand pushed me to reorient the assemblages of transporting items to and from my home, like many others. Plastic bags now seem entirely ridiculous and unnecessary. But this final step did not happen without a collective push from public institutions. In the same way, pioneering feminists' reorienting their domestic relationships in the home eventually led to widespread changes in law and policy that supported greater gender equality, even for those who were not activists. I think this is what Ruha Benjamin means by viral justice: small seeds of world-making work that spread and proliferate in much the same way as viruses do.[3] I take some hope and inspiration from these stories while often feeling utterly downcast by the many things that have not changed. As humans in more-than-human collectives and communities, the task in front of us is daunting.

For those of us in the most wasteful and environmentally disconnected societies of the world, the task is to rework our damaging modes of embodied hygiene that rely on disposable and plastic products, large amounts of water, and large amounts of landfill space. These assemblages must shift. However, the task of shifting such assemblages requires a reworking of our very habits—habits that are embodied and embedded in ourselves, our homes, our infrastructure, and our societies. To shift assemblages requires collective effort and intentionality. It is not enough for me personally to refuse plastic bottles of shampoo, to teach my daughters to use menstrual cups, or to use infant toileting with my babies. It is not enough for you to switch to cloth nappies, not have children, install a composting toilet, or buy period panties. We might feel ethically superior to our neighbors in those actions, but as Nie Yuntai reminds us, guarding life must include the community and the moral and ethical ties that bind us together. But it is also not enough to give money to development agencies to install "proper" sanitation in Bangladesh, to teach nomadic Tibetan women to wash their hands, or to install beautiful, brand-new flush toilets in houses unconnected to the overloaded sewage system in Bhutan. Such actions might lead to some change against global indicators for sanitation, but neither leads to a deeper learning and engagement with better-adapted hygiene assemblages.

What comes next, then, for a postdevelopment politics of hygiene? This book has been structured around a series of collective actions, visible in the chapter titles. The actions that might be collectively taken, in our wider hybrid collectives of researcher and layperson, human and nonhuman, majority and minority world, include thinking multiplicity, holding out, shifting assemblages, traveling practices, and reassembling hygienes, all in the service of guarding life. Thinking multiplicity requires us to hold ourselves open to the possibilities of others; it requires us to look for the diversity of hygienes already present in the places we find ourselves, as well as in places further afield. Holding out is an action of salvaging and retaining those practices that are valuable and under threat by homogenizing forces. Shifting assemblages recognizes the trajectories of change present in our lives, often manifesting as universals in hygiene, medicine, and the body, but also the shadow assemblages of hygiene that are retained alongside these more normative practices. Traveling practices is the deliberate traveling or movement and adaptation of appropriate practices from one place to another. Reassembling hygienes is an act of intentional collective action for hygiene change built on lay research and experimentation in changing embodied habits. Finally, what is guarding life? It is the care-full and nuanced gathering of such actions in the interest of holistic wellbeing for all forms of life—microbes, qi, water cycles, decomposition cycles, bodies in both disease and health, other species, and more.

J. K. Gibson-Graham, in *A Postcapitalist Politics,* identify three forms of politics at work in shifting our economies to more just and sustainable assemblages: a politics of language, a politics of the subject, and a politics of collective action. A politics of language includes recognizing the performativity of language and the need for a language open to possibilities. I see this politics of language further articulated in the idea of thinking multiplicity that this book has detailed, as well as in the rereading of China's shifting assemblages and hygiene histories to show multiplicity. For Gibson-Graham, a politics of the subject includes recognizing the resistances and affective bonds that subjects had to previous forms of economy, and the need for new forms of affect and swerve in the bodies and minds of economic subjects in postcapitalist community economies. I see this politics of the subject further articulated in the deeply embodied explorations of this book in the practices of holding out and intentionally traveling practices of hygiene. Finally, a politics of collective action includes developing new ways to be collectives through participatory action research, which this book has further articulated through development of hybrid collectives experimenting with and caring for new hygienes. Just as Gibson-Graham move beyond the strictures of analyzing capitalism alone to begin to think of postcapitalism, this book has sought to delink hygiene thinking from

Westernized development, thus opening up the question of what guarding life might look like for all of us, wherever we are.

As Stephen Healy notes, the difficulty in reworking ourselves for a new mode of humanity is that it is not only different ways of thinking and organizing and doing things that we must pay attention to, but also different ways of being in the world. This way of being requires us to live in common.[4] Many of us are out of practice. Many of us have become accustomed to a one-world world where knowledge is formalized, contained, homogenized, and distributed. This system has certainly failed in my home country of Aotearoa New Zealand, however, where sanitation infrastructures and water quality have not been adequately cared for under the world-leading legislation and engineering systems of the colonial state, and where commercialized hygiene and cleaning products continue to wreak havoc with both wastewater and landfill. What is required of us now is the ability to proliferate the multiple, experimental, place-based, and diverse ways of doing and being, and to increase the capacity to act differently, rather than doubling down on the Great Singularity.[5] It is not a simple task, but it is one I am more certain of day by day.

POSTSCRIPT: BEGINNINGS AND ENDINGS

In one sense, I finish this book the way I began some ten years ago: in a place of not knowing. I do not know much about the kinds of possibilities out there for different hygiene futures. I do not know what this new Earth era holds for us or our children, or the Earth others who survive alongside us. I began with little more than a desire to "imagine and work out new ways to live with the Earth," to contribute to the aforementioned different mode of humanity.[6] I began with the hope that things can be different, because already, right now, multiple contemporaneous realities offer us difference, options, glimmers of hope, and collective care subjectivities. I began with an attempt to see and think through those multiple possibilities by using strategies outside the tired, old colonizing teleologies of modernization and development. I began with a faith that the possibilities already present could somehow help me to imagine (and enact) an uncertain, hopeful, and experimental decolonizing, postdevelopment hygiene project. These hopes, desires, attempts, and faith are now better articulated and informed, but they have not changed much. In fact, I have come to appreciate the possibilities latent in a place of not knowing, because this is where new thinking and change can happen.[7]

In another sense, I finish this book a long way from where I began. I began as a heavily pregnant twenty-five-year-old, arriving in Australia to complete a degree with quite a different project in mind. I had little idea as to how my husband and I would manage our work and studies and writing around caring for babies and children and community. However, during this project, I lived in five different cities in three different countries, birthing four children in three different places. Xiao Shi, head nurse Zhang, and the venerable grannies who coached me have all seen their charges grow up; like them, I soon will watch my first charge, my daughter, leave home. The changes in hygiene practice since then have been encouraging: while the 500 mothers on OzNappyfree have slipped away from that forum, the Facebook EC group in Aotearoa New Zealand has 796 members, and there are at least two in the United States with 8,000-plus members in each. One in the United Kingdom has 8,600. A global group has 20,689 members. In the subway train in Boston, I saw an advertisement for period underwear. My local pharmacy in Christchurch sells menstrual cups. There are cloth nappies in the supermarket near my in-laws' house. Infant disposable nappy companies continue to despair at the low penetration of the products into Chinese markets. I do not really know how much I contributed to the proliferation of these knowledges—or even whether my research contributed, because they are certainly the result of wider collective actions. But my engagement with these practices and groups has certainly changed me.

Isn't this how change happens—starting with what we have, then moving forward? I have come to embrace the restrictions and possibilities alike of my own position as an academic, parent, and cross-cultural thinker; and have begun to work out what I can do here and now, with what I have to offer. I do not mean to say that the world needs more academics (it most likely does not), but it does need more caring hybrid research collectives experimenting for change. I do not mean that the world needs more babies (it arguably does not), but it does need more of the softness and awareness that learning to be affected by babies brings. I do not mean that the world needs more cosmopolitans skipping around the globe in blissful ignorance of their jet fuel use (once again, it does not), but it does need more of the edge-walking sense of other ways of doing things to which a postdevelopment, cross-cultural engagement can inspire. In coming to think about Plumwood's call for different modes of humanity, I have had to think about what it might mean to fully be human myself, with others, to find ways to care for the commons in the places I find myself, sometimes involuntarily.

Finally, my own children have been essential partners in changing me; we have together traveled a path of communication, connection, experimentation, and embodied knowing. Who knows what the future holds for them, and for our planet? I hope they can continue to partner with others in guarding planetary life in all its vibrant, diverse forms—and, of course, continue to wash properly behind their ears.

Acknowledgments

As will no doubt be clear from the text of this book, my research and writing endeavors have not been carried out alone. While many people have contributed to the larger project from which this book emerges, some special people have been particularly significant. First thanks go to my editor at the University of Minnesota Press, Jason Weidemann, and series editors Katherine Gibson, Stephen Healy, Maliha Safri, and Kevin St. Martin for sticking with me for so long. Thanks also to Caitlin Baird, Mona-Lynn Courteau, and Mike Stoffel, who contributed editorial support at different stages. This has made the book better than it would have been otherwise. Thanks to Junxi Qian of Hong Kong University for providing the phrase "caring for life" for the title. This is an alternative translation for *weisheng,* hygiene, that connects nicely to my interest in care in this book.

For inspiration and mentorship throughout the many years of this project, I thank Katherine Gibson and Gerda Roelvink. Katherine took me on despite my late stage of pregnancy and provided a solid intellectual grounding in community economies and feminist economic geography, shaping both the initial work that became this book and commenting on the final drafts. As the joint authorial presence comprising J. K. Gibson-Graham, Katherine and Julie inspired me to believe that things could indeed be different, and that I had a role in enacting this difference. Gerda's intellectual work and her careful and attentive comments on my first rehearsals of these arguments have indelibly shaped my ongoing scholarship in a multitude of important ways.

For quiet, ongoing encouragement for many years, I thank Katharine McKinnon. My thinking is very much influenced by our shared work and conversations since she first encouraged me to consider doctoral research and introduced me to the Community Economies Collective. For generous engagement throughout the process of preparing and refining the book, I thank Stephen Healy. He was an endlessly encouraging discussion partner, read and gave comments on the entire book in less than a week, and revealed an amazing ability to connect the dots between my work and everything else going on in the social sciences (and more often, the mysteries of the universe).

Other members of the Community Economies Collective have been important in this work. Gradon Diprose has helped me refine and clarify my thinking around how social change happens in our shared work in Aotearoa. Many hours of assemblage discussion with Ann Hill informed and refined the ideas in this book. Jenny Cameron's work on learning to be affected has continued to inspire me, and I have also benefited from her expertise in teaching writing as well as her detailed review of the book. The Community Economies Collective continues to provide me with an intellectual home base from which I can make my forays into the world of scholarship. Thanks to all those not mentioned who continue to make this possible. I was able to spend time in Bolsena, Italy, on a Julie Graham Community Economies Research Fellowship in 2017 and 2018 while writing this book. A Rutherford Fellowship from the Royal Society of New Zealand enabled the final push to submission. Funding from the Australian National University enabled fieldwork in China in 2006, 2007, and 2009, with support from Qinghai Nationalities University. Macquarie University, Hong Kong Polytechnic University, and Peking University supported other visits in 2012 and 2013. Funding from an Erskine Fellowship at the University of Canterbury enabled a visit in 2018.

In Xining, many women whom I cannot name here supported and challenged me as I grew to understand and experience life in the city. The members of OzNappyfree and Ecommunic8anz provided not just insights into elimination communication but also friendship and support as I transitioned into parenthood. There are others who have commented on parts of this book, supported me institutionally, or contributed to getting it done in various ways: Amy Sun Xiao Fei, Bethan Greener, the Braun family, Deirdre Hart, David Conradson, Eric Pawson, the Foggin family, Glenn Banks, Helen Po Ping Nian, Helen Sturgeon, Helena Bai, Lu Zimei and family, Ma Shengmei, Ma Xiaolong, Marnie Holmes, Michelle Bland, Mona-Lynn Courteau, Nina Muijsson, Peyman Zawar-Reza, Rebecca Mottram,

Rebecca Poh, Regina Scheyvens, Robyn Longhurst, Rosemary and Dan Joyce, and Sophie Ma. Many thanks to you all. Over the years, doctoral students have drawn attention to aspects of this work that need refining or are most valuable to retain, especially Amba Sepie, Anmeng Liu, Chemi Zhuoga, Huong Thi Do, Ririn Haryani, S. M. Waliuzzaman, Tingting Zhang, and Tsehua Dorji.

Finally, my own family has patiently endured my long work hours during some intense periods I spent writing this book, and over the past decade has followed me to conferences, fieldwork, and new jobs without complaint. I thank my parents, Nick and Janmarie Hoskins, for giving me a solid start to life, toilet training me, and washing all those nappies. I thank my husband, Travis Dombroski, for some twenty years of companionship, as well as his support in making this book possible, particularly his attentive care of our four children. I thank Casimir for reconnecting me to the embodied work of caring for babies once again, Emmaus for his curious questions and fun propositions for breaks, Analiese for years of wonderful, affectionate, and encouraging cards and drawings, and Imogen for being the baby with whom it all started—as well as the wonderful teen she has become. I hope in turn I have made some small difference in the world that you will all grow up in.

Notes

INTRODUCTION

1. Plumwood, "Review." See also Plumwood, *Environmental Culture,* for more on her thinking.

2. "Out of the way" is a term I have adopted from Anna Tsing, with thanks to Yvonne Underhill-Sem for drawing it to my attention. It is a useful term for thinking about how some places of the world are frequently overlooked. See Tsing, *In the Realm of the Diamond Queen;* and Underhill-Sem, "Marked Bodies."

3. For surviving well, see Gibson-Graham, Cameron, and Healy, *Take Back the Economy;* Dombroski, Duojie, and McKinnon, "Surviving Well"; McKinnon, Healy, and Dombroski, "Surviving Well Together." For survivance, see the works of Gerald Vizenor, particularly *Native Liberty.* See also the special issue "Survivance" of *E-Flux Architecture:* Axel, Hirsch, and Therrien, "Editorial—Survivance." For flourishing and the idea of sustainability as flourishing, see Ehrenfeld and Hoffman, *Flourishing.* For more-than-human wellbeing, see Yates, Dombroski, and Dionisio, "Dialogues for Wellbeing." In the final edits of this book, I also became interested in Ruha Benjamin's concept of viral justice, which has a lot of crossover with all these concepts as well as an overlapping prefigurative politics; see Benjamin, *Viral Justice.*

4. Rogaski, *Hygienic Modernity;* Lei, "Moral Community."

5. In April 2020, near the end of a strict preemptive lockdown, a nationwide poll revealed that 87 percent of New Zealanders supported the government's response—an unprecedented level of support for a government policy that restricted all movement, apart from essential workers and trips to purchase food or short periods of outdoor exercise.

6. Dombroski, "Multiplying Possibilities."

7. It also included Australians and New Zealanders living in other parts of the world, such as myself.

8. My research went through ethical approval processes at the Australian National University, where I was a PhD student at the time. I amended the ethics by adding

the online case study and developing protocols of ethnographic research on this virtual forum. I received permission from the moderator to post about the research project in late 2008, and the group discussed my project and whether they wanted to be involved. I began collecting posts from January 1, 2009, and finished December 31, 2009. In 2015, I conducted a follow-up series of email interviews and collected responses from previous participants about how their hygiene practices had changed over the intervening years. I also asked for written reflections from members on the OzNappyfree Facebook group and the Aotearoa New Zealand Elimination Communication Facebook group, but I did not receive any. This follow-up research received ethics approval from the University of Canterbury human ethics committee. See Dombroski, "Learning to Be Affected."

9. See particularly Dombroski, "Hybrid Activist Collectives."

10. Larsen and Johnson, *Being Together in Place.*

11. For a "politics of possibilities," see Gibson-Graham, *Postcapitalist Politics;* for "making other worlds possible," see Roelvink, St. Martin, and Gibson-Graham, *Making Other Worlds Possible;* for "dignified worlds," see Roelvink, *Building Dignified Worlds.*

1. THINKING MULTIPLICITY

1. My understanding of assemblages is most heavily influenced by John Law's work, where I first encountered the idea in the early 2000s. It immediately made sense to me and provided a language for how I understood the world and the patterns of materialities, spatialities, and socialities therein. The assemblage thinking that has descended more directly from Deleuze has also been part of my wider networks of thinking; however, the accessibility of Law's work means my imagination returns there most frequently. See in particular Law, *After Method.*

2. I have written about this in more depth in Dombroski, "Multiplying Possibilities."

3. Jewitt, "Geographies of Shit."

4. Iossifova, "Urban (Sanitation) Transformation."

5. Hashemi, "Sanitation Sustainability Index."

6. Iossifova, "Urban (Sanitation) Transformation."

7. Jewitt, "Geographies of Shit"; Iossifova, "Urban (Sanitation) Transformation."

8. See the life cycle assessment and assumptions made by O'Brien et al., "Life Cycle Assessment."

9. Paddison, "Reuse? Compost? Dump?"

10. Dombroski, "What Other Countries Can Teach Us."

11. Jewitt, "Geographies of Shit," 610.

12. Iossifova, "Urban (Sanitation) Transformation."

13. See Longhurst, "(Dis)embodied Geographies"; and Longhurst, *Bodies.*

14. Black and Fawcett call it the *Last Taboo,* but they do not theorize it in any significant way. Others, such as Robyn Longhurst, have drawn on the work of Elizabeth Grosz and Julia Kristeva to think more about how patriarchal masculine ways of being in the world tend to emphasize hard-and-fast boundaries and exhibit disgust at the leakiness and soft boundaries of bodies, and women's bodies in particular. When this

way of thinking dominates without recognizing other modes of thinking and being, it is called masculinist. See Longhurst, *Bodies;* Grosz, *Volatile Bodies;* and Kristeva, *Powers of Horror.*

15. Shove, *Comfort,* 20.

16. Shove, *Comfort,* 20.

17. Shove, "Social Theory."

18. Global Public–Private Partnership for Handwashing, *Handwashing Handbook,* 5.

19. This is even though around the time of the interview with the pediatrician, diarrhea and respiratory tract infections were not the biggest killers of children in Qinghai. According to Rudan et al., "Causes of Deaths," causes of death for Qinghai children under five, in order of importance, are as follows: "other"; birth asphyxia; pneumonia; preterm birth complications; accidents; congenital abnormality; sudden infant death syndrome; diarrhea; and neonatal infant sepsis. Pneumonia (a respiratory tract infection) is certainly significant, but because it is also related to exposure, handwashing for plateau dwellers may not have the preventative effect it has been shown to have elsewhere. We must keep in mind, however, that the reliability of death reporting in Qinghai is not high; see Zeng et al., "Measuring the Completeness."

20. "Hygiene," *Oxford English Dictionary,* www.oed.com. See also Rogaski, *Hygienic Modernity.*

21. See, e.g., patient education advice such as Medscape's "Frostbite," www.e medicine.medscape.com. My scientist colleagues who regularly travel to do fieldwork in the dry valleys of Antarctica also inform me handwashing is not a good idea.

22. Ashenburg, *The Dirt on Clean.*

23. Xu et al., "Understanding Land Use."

24. I also think of the devastating interactions between colonizers and Indigenous populations in the Americas, Australia, New Zealand, and the Pacific, where previously unknown diseases decimated populations after contact.

25. Kedgely, *Mum's the Word;* Smith, *Clean.*

26. The hydatid worm is ingested accidentally after contact with dog feces, causing cysts in the internal organs of its host, which are difficult to remove and can cause death.

27. See, e.g., Li et al., "Widespread Co-endemicity."

28. Bai et al., "Survey on Cystic Echinococcosis."

29. See analysis in Esteva, "Development."

30. See Escobar, "Development, Violence."

31. Kothari, "From Colonialism to Development."

32. Klein and Morreo, *Postdevelopment.*

33. Esteva and Escobar, "Post-development @ 25."

34. Law, "What's Wrong."

35. Law discusses the differences between perspectivist approaches to reality and those that truly recognize other ontologies and epistemologies; see Law, *After Method.*

36. Zoe Todd writes of this eloquently in a 2016 essay reflecting on a lecture from Bruno Latour: "Again, I thought with a sinking feeling in my chest, it appeared that another Euro-Western academic narrative, in this case the trendy and dominant

Ontological Turn (and/or posthumanism, and/or cosmopolitics—all three of which share tangled roots, and can be mobilised distinctly or collectively, depending on who you ask), and discourses of how to organise ourselves around and communicate with the constituents of complex and contested world(s) (or multiverses, if you're into the whole brevity thing)—was spinning itself on the backs of non-European thinkers. . . . No, here we were celebrating and worshipping a European thinker for 'discovering,' or newly articulating by drawing on a European intellectual heritage, what many an Indigenous thinker around the world could have told you for millennia." Todd, "Indigenous Feminist's Take," 7.

37. Here I'm thinking of Anna Tsing's *Friction*. There are many more.

38. All of Anna Tsing's work is relevant, but I'm particularly thinking here of *In the Realm of the Diamond Queen, Friction,* and *The Mushroom at the End of the World.*

39. Adams et al., "Having a 'Safe Delivery.'"

40. Liu, *Otherness of Self.*

41. Massey, *For Space,* 5. See her wonderful discussion throughout.

42. In fact, Thomassen called it "the multiple modernities paradigm," considering it to be "an extremely influential approach in anthropology." See Thomassen, "Anthropology and Its Many Modernities," 160.

43. Escobar, "Beyond the Third World," 225.

44. See Escobar, *Designs.*

45. De Sousa Santos, "WSF," 241. See also Gibson-Graham, "Surplus Possibilities," which makes an argument for postdevelopment as a practice of possibility as well as critique.

46. See, e.g., the whole 2022 volume of the journal *Sustainability Science,* including Kaul et al., "Alternatives." See also Kothari et al., *Pluriverse;* Dinerstein and Deneulin, "Hope Movements"; Escobar and Harcourt, "Post-development Possibilities"; Escobar and Jeong, "Postdevelopment"; and McGregor, "New Possibilities?"

47. Puig de la Bellacasa, *Matters of Care.*

48. McKinnon, "Geopolitics of Birth," 3.

49. McKinnon, "Geopolitics of Birth," 3.

50. For these actual examples, see McKinnon, Healy, and Dombroski, "Surviving Well Together."

51. Butler, *Gender Trouble.*

52. Mol, *Body Multiple,* 43.

53. Mol, *Body Multiple,* 44.

54. Mol, *Body Multiple,* 55.

55. Rogaski, *Hygienic Modernity.*

56. Lei, *Neither Donkey nor Horse.* I have drawn on many of Lei's pieces in other journals and books as well; these will be cited more specifically in chapter 3.

57. See, e.g., Leung and Furth, *Health and Hygiene in Chinese East Asia.* This edited volume includes the work of Warwick Anderson, Charlotte Furth, Sean Hsiang-lin Lei, Angela Leung, Ruth Rogaski, Wu Chia-ling, and Yu Xinzhong.

58. See Iossifova, "Everyday Practices"; Iossifova, "Urban (Sanitation) Transformation"; and Liu, Browne, and Iossifova, "Socio-material Approach."

59. Smith, *Clean;* Douglas, *Purity and Danger;* Campkin and Cox, *Dirt;* Curtis and Biran, "Dirt, Disgust, and Disease"; Grosz, *Volatile Bodies;* Lahiri-Dutt, "Medicalising Menstruation"; Longhurst, *Bodies;* Jewitt, "Geographies of Shit."

60. See, e.g., Black and Fawcett, *Last Taboo.*

61. Vandegrift et al., "Cleanliness in Context."

62. I did not find much evidence that it helped scientists question hygiene practices. A promising-looking study by university scientists on the effects of Chinese postpartum practices on the microbiome persisted in labeling women as having "poor hygiene" when they were following culturally prescribed practices. See Wang et al., "Effect of Maternal Postpartum Practices."

63. Rogaski, *Hygienic Modernity.*

64. Law, *After Method,* 41.

65. Massey, *For Space,* 9.

66. For a critique of strong constructionism, see Haraway, "Situated Knowledges."

67. Law, *After Method,* 42.

68. Haraway, "Situated Knowledges," 579.

69. Tsing, *Friction.*

2. HOLDING OUT

1. DeVries and deVries, "Cultural Relativity."

2. Rogoff, *Cultural Nature.*

3. *Ba* (把) refers to the action of grasping the child under the legs. *Niao* (尿) refers to urine or urinating. Some student translators assisting me with my transcripts translated *baniao* rather cumbersomely as "holding the baby's legs apart so it can urinate."

4. For assisted infant toileting, see Sun and Rugolotto, "Assisted Infant Toilet Training." For elimination communication, see Bender and She, "Elimination Communication." For natural infant hygiene, see Bauer, *Diaper Free!*

5. Open-crotch pants are similar to split-crotch pants, but with a much larger cutaway area at the back.

6. Although some boutique baby shops in Xining sold Japanese-made *niaobu* equivalents alongside leakproof nappy covers, none of the women I saw ever used anything but homemade *niaobu*.

7. There is no tradition of plastic nappy covers in China, for reasons that will become clear.

8. As I will discuss in more detail later, Australian and New Zealand mothers tend to respond with breastfeeding first, then to unsettledness with elimination-related interactions, leading to a different sort of infant toileting practice.

9. The Hui people are a Muslim group, many of whom descend from Persian traders. In 2011, there were approximately 10.5 million people registered as Hui in China. Hui Muslims have recently come under pressure to resist Arab influences in their religious practice. See Feng, "China Is Removing Domes."

10. China's one-child policy did not apply equally to all. In 2009, rural dwellers could have a second child if the first is a girl; minority people were entitled to one

extra child (so two children in the city or three in the countryside); and if neither parent has any siblings, the couple was entitled to two children. In 2016, China shifted to a two-child policy, and in 2021 to a three-child policy. The fertility rate continues to fall; in 2022, it is now estimated to be 1.3, down from 1.6 in 2016. In 2009, it was around 1.8 across the country. In Xining in 2009, mothers reported that if they were under thirty, they must ensure a four-year gap between children—that is, one child must be toilet independent before the next child is born. In 2021, the one-child policy was replaced with a three-child policy along with a suite of support measures introduced to encourage a higher fertility rate. The results of these policies remain to be seen, but in general, couples are already reluctant to have larger families. See Yang et al., "China's Fertility Change." See also Attané, "Trois enfants pour tous en Chine?"

11. In fact, the company chose not to translate the name Pampers into Chinese because the word has a negative connotation of raising a spoiled child. The brand is known as *bang bao shi* (邦宝适). *Bang bao* suggests supporting someone or helping with something precious, and *shi* refers to disposable nappies.

12. Frazier, "How P&G Brought the Diaper Revolution to China."

13. See Fair Companies' website at www.faircompanies.com.

14. Minchin, "Infant Formula: A Mass, Uncontrolled Trial in Perinatal Care."

15. Landbank Consultancy, report prepared for the Women's Environmental Network (WEN), "A Review of Procter and Gamble's Environmental Balances for Disposable and Reusable Nappies," 1991, Archives and Manuscripts, National Childbirth Trust, Wellcome Collection, London, wellcomecollection.org/works/z9tcmh 64.

16. Mothering, "Politics of Diapers."

17. A life cycle analysis tries to account for the environmental impact of the product from manufacture and raw materials to disposal and breakdown of discarded product. For further discussion of problems with the methods used in these studies of disposable nappies, see What a Waste at www.whatawaste.info. For the environment agency report, see Aumonier, Collins, and Garrett, *Update Lifecycle Assessment Study.*

18. Environment Agency report: Aumônier, Collins, and Garrett, *Update Lifecycle Assessment Study.* Australian study: O'Brien et al., "Life Cycle Assessment."

19. Notten, Gower, and Lewis, "Single-Use Nappies." See also a more recent overview study: Płotka-Wasylka et al., "End-of-Life Management."

20. Aggravation of asthma: Anderson and Anderson, "Acute Respiratory Effects." Chemical nappy rashes: *Child Health Alert,* "Diaper Rash." Urinary tract dysfunction: Bakker and Wyndaele, "Changes in the Toilet Training of Children." Research links the delay in toilet training to a change in attitudes, but there is also some evidence to suggest this attitude change has been enabled by the widespread availability and convenience of disposable nappies; see Bakker, van Gool, and Wyndaele, "Results of a Questionnaire."

21. Narain, "Mother, 25, Reunited."

22. Frazier, "How P&G Brought the Diaper Revolution to China."

23. Frazier, "How P&G Brought the Diaper Revolution to China."

24. Ruth Rogaski quotes an ancient formula for *weisheng* that encourages health seekers to concoct a tonic that uses young boys' urine, among other medicinal substances. See Rogaski, *Hygienic Modernity.*

25. Some research in other areas of China indicates that the deformity referred to is most likely rickets and could in fact be caused by various postpartum practices like not eating vegetables and not going outdoors into the sunlight. Historically, many families tried to prevent this through swaddling practices, which have largely been discontinued; see Strand et al., "Doing the Month."

26. For the Pampers scandal, see Wohl, "P&G Faces Growing Backlash."

27. Flaws, *Handbook.*

28. Dunn, "Nappywars."

29. See, e.g., Schum et al., "Sequential Acquisition."

30. Largo et al., "Development"; Sillén, "Bladder Function."

31. I found some research that supports an earlier development. Unsurprisingly, it is all from research teams that include researchers with Chinese names. See Yeung et al., "Some New Insights"; and Liu et al., "Attaining Nocturnal Urinary Control."

INTERLUDE: THE BODY MULTIPLE

1. The quotes in this interlude come from a translated transcription of the recorded interview. The transcription was completed by three student research assistants from Qinghai Minorities University. The translation was drafted by students in the translation program at Macquarie University, and I revised it directly from the recordings. In some places I represent the participant's actual transcribed words in poetic form to illustrate the rhythm of her speech.

3. SHIFTING ASSEMBLAGES

1. Massey, *For Space,* 151.

2. Rogaski, *Hygienic Modernity.*

3. Lei, "Habituating Individuality"; Lei, "Sovereignty and the Microscope"; Lei, *Neither Donkey nor Horse;* Lei, "Moral Community."

4. Tsing, *Friction.*

5. Liu, *Mirage of China,* viii.

6. Biomedical researchers have found relationships between hormones and breast milk letdown and production as well as links between emotional states and hormones, particularly during birth. See Dixon, Skinner, and Foureur, "Emotional and Hormonal Pathways." This idea is not so widespread in breastfeeding support or biomedical training, however, and it usually understands hormones as causing emotions, not the other way around.

7. Men and Guo, *General Introduction to Traditional Chinese Medicine.*

8. For a full discussion of this, see Rogaski, *Hygienic Modernity.*

9. Veith, "Introduction."

10. Chen and Swartzman, "Health Beliefs," 391.

11. As cited and translated in Men and Guo, *General Introduction to Traditional Chinese Medicine,* 71.

12. See Men and Guo, *General Introduction to Traditional Chinese Medicine;* and Veith, "Introduction."

13. Pillsbury, "Doing the Month."

14. Rogaski, *Hygienic Modernity,* 31.

15. Rogaski, *Hygienic Modernity,* 29.

16. Rogaski, *Hygienic Modernity,* 29. See also chapter 1.

17. This quotation is from the complete works of Zhang Jingyue (1624). Zhang, *Complete Compendium.* Many thanks to Sue Cochrane of Western Sydney University for passing this on to me.

18. Even in biomedical research, stress hormones can come through breast milk, although it has not been shown to affect infant crying, an indicator of unsettledness. See Hechler et al., "Are Cortisol Concentrations."

19. Ruth Rogaski's chapter entitled "Conquering the One Hundred Diseases" is a survey of texts on *weisheng* published before the twentieth century. See Rogaski, *Hygienic Modernity.*

20. Rogaski, *Hygienic Modernity,* 44.

21. Farquhar, *Way of Life.*

22. Lei, "Sovereignty and the Microscope."

23. See Angela Leung's work on the evolution of the idea of *chuanran* over the course of different periods in history. For Leung, "the term *chuanran* reflects how Chinese medicine easily accommodated pluralistic models of events, including outbreaks of disease, imagining them as the outcome of a dynamically interacting web of influences." Leung, "Evolution," 43.

24. Rogaski, *Hygienic Modernity,* 83.

25. Snowden, *Epidemics and Society,* 49.

26. Luesink, "Introduction."

27. Tianjin is nowhere near Xining, where I did my fieldwork. However, Rogaski's account is widely recognized as the best study on the rise of hygiene and public health in China. The history of the northwest is dominated by warlords, most famously Ma Bufang, a Muslim warlord who later became governor and then ambassador to Saudi Arabia. There is further historical work to be done on hygiene and *weisheng* discourses in Qinghai province and the northwest more generally. One study discusses immunization in Gansu, a nearby northwestern province, in the republican period, although it also draws on Rogaski's work for context; see Brazelton, "Frontiers of Immunology."

28. Rogaski, *Hygienic Modernity,* 84.

29. Green, Carrillo, and Betancourt, "Why the Disease-Based Model of Medicine Fails Our Patients."

30. See Clarke et al., "Biomedicalization."

31. McKinnon, *Birthing Work.* Dombroski, McKinnon, and Healy, "Beyond the Birth Wars."

32. For example, many women are prescribed antibiotics while giving birth as a preventative measure, especially if *Streptococcus* is found in a vaginal swab. See Schafer and Phillippi, "Group B Streptococcal Bacteriuria."

33. See, for example, the history of evidence around delayed cord clamping. Immediate cord clamping after birth was introduced without evidence. Randomized control trials were eventually able to show that delayed cord clamping was beneficial for both babies and mothers in normal circumstances; see Committee on Obstetric Practice, "Timing of Umbilical Cord Clamping." See also research on the "cascade of interventions" that begins with epidural analgesia or artificial rupture of membranes: Fox et al., "Response to: The 'Cascade of Interventions.'"

34. McKinnon, "Geopolitics of Birth."

35. The ultimate biomedicalization has been visible in the data gathering and policy making around hygiene during the Covid-19 pandemic, with large-scale, population-level interventions based on data collected and reported daily.

36. Robinson, *Cross-Cultural Child Development*.

37. Youkee and Graham-Harrison, "Miracle, Miracle."

38. Karasik et al., "Ties that Bind."

39. The WHO multicenter growth reference study collected primary growth data (www.who.int). However, one part of the study still used six "universal" milestones as its starting point that were gleaned from a North American study, which included crawling.

40. Tsing, *Friction*, 7.

41. Tsing, *Friction*.

42. See Yang, "From Discourse of Weakness." The discourse came to light again in 2020, when the *Wall Street Journal* published an article on Covid-19 calling China the real "sick man of Asia." Three *Wall Street Journal* journalists were subsequently deported from China in retaliation. Elaine Yau of the *South China Morning Post* revisits the history of the term; see Yau, "China Enraged."

43. Yang, "From Discourse of Weakness."

44. See Hong, *Footbinding, Feminism, and Freedom;* and Lei, "Moral Community."

45. The fact that Meiji elites and translator Nagayo Sensei recognized the interconnected practices of medicine, technology, and policing as significant in many ways prefigures the work of Foucault on biopower in Europe, as Rogaski points out in her introduction to *Hygienic Modernity*.

46. Lei, "Moral Community."

47. Liu quoted in Lei, "Moral Community," 477.

48. Chen translated by and quoted in Lei, "Moral Community," 477.

49. Rogaski, *Hygienic Modernity*, 1.

50. Tan, "Plague Fighter."

51. Lei, "Sovereignty and the Microscope."

52. Lynteris, "Plague Masks"; Yan, "What Can and Can't Be Learned."

53. Yu, "Masks and Geopolitics"; Lei, "Sovereignty and the Microscope." See also the image collections of Richard Pearson at Harvard University and of Wu Tien-Leh at the National University of Singapore.

54. Tan, "Plague Fighter."

55. He was nominated for a Nobel Prize in medicine in 1935; see the nomination archive at www.nobelprize.org.

56. Tan, "Plague Fighter."

57. Since I began researching and teaching the story of Dr. Wu in 2010, the discourse has changed dramatically. The Covid-19 pandemic has brought renewed attention to Dr. Wu's story and the pandemic measures put in place. Many journalists based in the United States have used the story as an opportunity to show the importance of masks and quarantine measures, presenting a romanticized view of what was a chaotic and catastrophic time. While it is nothing new to use history to make an important contemporary point, I have tried to focus on academic articles with good historical citations.

58. Lei, *Neither Donkey nor Horse*, 8.

59. Hsu, "History of Chinese Medicine"; Lei, *Neither Donkey nor Horse*.

60. Lei, *Neither Donkey nor Horse*, 9.

61. Lei, *Neither Donkey nor Horse*.

62. Hsu, "History of Chinese Medicine."

63. Here she quotes Qu Qiubai, a May Fourth thinker who argued that China could "catch up" with the West. These arguments were being made by a wide range of intellectuals, industrialists, and thinkers at this time, well before they were given political power in the Great Leap Forward in the late 1960s. See Shih, *Lure,* 49.

64. Massey, *For Space,* 5.

65. According to Sanchun Xu and Danian Hu, the integration was primarily for economic reasons. The barefoot doctors started off using mainly Western biomedicine, but they switched to TCM when resources were scarce. It was the main method by which Western biomedicine was introduced to rural China, in partnership with TCM. See Xu and Hu, "Barefoot Doctors."

66. Wind damage is an important concept in TCM that explains a susceptibility to pernicious external influences on health when yin and yang are imbalanced. See Dashtdar et al., "Concept of Wind."

67. Sedgwick, *Tendencies,* 6.

68. Lei, "Moral Community," 496. Other texts also show that during this time, Nie wrote many repudiations of Christianity and was involved in collaborations with other Buddhist thinkers seeking to question the role of science in the new China. See Sun, "Apostate Nie Yuntai's Comparison"; Zheng and Fan, "Wealth Lies in Virtue"; and Hammerstrom, "Buddhist Critique."

69. Nie cited in Lei, "Moral Community," 497.

70. Although Lei does not draw on diverse economies thinking when reading for difference—see, e.g., Gibson-Graham, "Reading for Economic Difference"—I see many parallels in his attention to the things that do not add up and to the rich junctures where everything does not have to mean the same thing (to paraphrase Sedgwick, *Tendencies,* 6). Instead, Lei reads the historical landscape of health and hygiene with an eye to difference, paying attention to the bits and pieces of information and ideas that tell a story other than the hygienic modernity story we have become familiar with. As Gibson-Graham, "Reading for Economic Difference," writes, reading for difference "is a thinking practice, a research method and an intervention in making

worlds" where those worlds might have possibility proliferated through the stories we tell (483).

71. Lei, "Moral Community," 479.

72. Lei, "Moral Community," 492.

73. Chinese custom holds that it is polite to urge others to eat before you, and to take only small amounts but continue to eat as your host urges you to. Serving yourself first and eating only once would disrupt the entire social and community dynamic of the eating ritual for the sake of one's own health.

74. Lei, "Habituating Individuality."

75. Lei, "Moral Community," 492.

76. Hammerstrom, "Buddhist Critique."

77. Lei, "Moral Community," 478.

78. Lei, "Moral Community," 478.

79. Here I draw on John Law's language and thinking in *After Method*.

80. For understanding the body in feminist politics as the "place closest in," see Harcourt, *Body Politics*, 23. For "articulations within," see Massey, *For Space*, 130.

81. I have written in more detail on this elsewhere; see Dombroski, "Seeing Diversity."

82. See Cheng, *"Taijiao,"* and note the unproblematized use of the term "eugenics" in *taijiao* thinking. Eugenics in China was certainly implied in much of the context of the work on child care, hygienic modernity, the "sick man of Asia," and modernization. As Chung writes, such thinking was behind the government push for Han relocation into minority areas for intermingling and intermarriage, apparently to strengthen national genetics and unity. However, the concept is prevalent in contemporary China as well as in both science and policy, as Chung's research shows. Chung, "Better Science."

4. TRAVELING PRACTICES

1. "Not a Joke," *New Zealand Herald*.

2. Ramaswamy, "Parents Toilet-Training Their Newborn Babies."

3. Das, "Mayim Bialik."

4. Dunn, "Nappywars."

5. Christie, "Toilet Training."

6. No justification is given why mothers are used as the unit of analysis rather than both parents.

7. Christie, "Toilet Training," 30.

8. Christie, "Toilet Training," 33.

9. People typed while breastfeeding often enough that the code "nak" was used to refer to "nursing at keyboard," signaling possible typing errors.

10. Bauer, *Diaper Free!;* Boucke, *Infant Potty Training;* Olson, *Go Diaper Free*.

11. Woolen blankets are put through a very hot machine wash, often with lanolin, which shrinks the wool and turns the blanket into a water-resistant felt surface.

12. Ekinsmyth, "Challenging the Boundaries."

13. See also the study by Yeung et al., "Some New Insights."

14. This was interesting to me, because in China, families had told me that there were many fruits that were not good foods for babies, who should be given easy-to-digest foods. Some Western nutritionists expressed frustration with this belief, but I suspect the effects of certain foods on digestion were simply better known in a culture where babies' elimination frequency is observed closely.

15. Here Amber used the "basically they do it when they are ready" line to defend her use of a parent-initiated pottying schedule. Interestingly, other part-time ECers used the same line to defend a more hands-off approach, because "they will start going (and getting out of nappies) when they are ready." Someone posted this same line with reference to an almost-five-year-old still in night nappies.

16. Except for the chapter in Mei-Ling Hopgood's *How Eskimos Keep Their Babies Warm and Other Adventures in Parenting.*

17. deVries and deVries, "Cultural Relativity."

18. As was also the case in the same period in New Zealand; see Kedgely, *Mum's the Word.*

19. deVries and deVries, "Cultural Relativity," 171.

20. deVries and deVries, "Cultural Relativity," 176.

21. deVries and deVries, "Cultural Relativity," 176.

22. See Wu, "Achieving Urinary Continence"; Wu, "Can Evidence-Based Medicine"; Duong, Jansson, and Hellström, "Vietnamese Mothers' Experiences"; and Sun and Rugolotto, "Assisted Infant Toilet Training."

23. Duong, Jansson, and Hellström, "Vietnamese Mothers' Experiences"; Duong et al., "Urinary Bladder Control."

24. "Attachment parenting" is a term coined by William and Martha Sears drawing on research into infant attachment extending back to John Bowlby's work on the emotional life of children; see, e.g., Sears and Sears, *Attachment Parenting Book.*

25. Even more child centered than attachment parenting, natural parenting draws on Jean Liedloff's 1986 book, *The Continuum Concept,* reflecting on her time living in the Amazon. It is a reinterpretation of babies and parents as primarily social mammals with a naturally evolved style of parenting based on instinct and preservation. It has been heavily critiqued by anthropologists and social scientists for its simplistic conclusions and understanding of what is natural.

26. Based on the rough and unscientific estimate of populations where EC-like practices (at least until recently) are the norm. Asia, Africa, and non-Anglo Oceania together have a population of more than five billion. Andrea Olson also claims that 50 percent of the world's population are toilet trained by age twelve months. See Olson, *Go Diaper Free.*

27. DeVries and deVries also make this point in "Cultural Relativity."

28. See the introduction to Tsing's *Friction* for more on this.

5. REASSEMBLING HYGIENES

1. Gibson-Graham, *Postcapitalist Politics,* 127.

2. "Swerve" here refers to Gibson-Graham's analysis of the film *The Full Monty.* The swerve is an embodied move, a failure of subjectification, where a different kind

of subject of possibility and joy was produced. See Gibson-Graham, *Postcapitalist Politics*.

3. Plumwood, "Ethics for Decolonisation," 1.

4. See Tsing, *Friction*.

5. This varies according to place and cultural background within Australia and New Zealand, of course, which both have multicultural populations. Even for dominant-Anglo heritage groups, I have found this type of behavior less appropriate, for example, in densely populated parts of Sydney. Also, in New Zealand, it is not unusual for people to go barefoot in public spaces, but this seems less common in Australia.

6. An obvious exception is in the prostrations of Tibetan Buddhism and some ancestor worship. This has meaning itself—humbling oneself through contact with the dirt. Hui/Islamic prayer generally includes a prayer mat, and the supplicants making prostrations in Tibetan Buddhist pilgrimages may wear protective coverings on the hands and knees. There are variations in what is imagined as dirty as well as variations in separation techniques. There are also geographical variations. What I describe here mostly relates to urban Xining.

7. Where Western-style toilets are present, children often learn to go over a bathroom drain until they are old enough to climb onto the toilet. In rural areas, homes often have nonflushing outhouse toilets, which may be little more than planks over a cesspit with holes cut to squat over. Because this is dangerous for small children, and because outhouses tend to be far away from the house, they may use alternatives for much longer.

8. Yu, "Treatment of Night Soil," 51.

9. Tsing, *Friction*.

10. Latour, "How to Talk about the Body?," 207.

11. Latour, "How to Talk about the Body?," 205.

12. Latour, "How to Talk about the Body?"

13. Cameron, Manhood, and Pomfrett, "Bodily Learning."

14. See the opening pages of Roelvink, *Building Dignified Worlds*.

15. Tronto, "There Is an Alternative."

16. See Cairns, "Organic Child"; and Cairns, Johnston, and MacKendrick, "Feeding the 'Organic Child.'"

17. Dombroski and Yates, "City as Laboratory."

18. See Dombroski et al., *Huritanga;* Dombroski and Yates, "City as Laboratory"; and Dombroski, Diprose, and Boles, "Can the Commons Be Temporary?"

19. See also Dombroski, "Hybrid Activist Collectives."

20. The main purpose of the forum was problem-solving when EC was not going well, so the most active threads were problem-based.

21. For research on this in the context of natural parenting in the United States, see Bobel, "Bounded Liberation" and "When Good Enough Isn't." My own experience of cloth nappy forums and Facebook groups informs my comment here too. People recited the correct way to wash nappies as proven by science to kill germs,

despite considerable possibilities for different washing techniques and a variety of parental goals. Killing germs might just be one! Convenience is certainly another.

22. See Latour and Woolgar, *Laboratory Life*.

23. See Farquhar and Lai, *Gathering Medicines*.

24. Callon and Rabeharisoa, "Research 'in the Wild.'"

25. Callon and Rabeharisoa, "Research 'in the Wild,'" 195.

26. Roelvink, "Collective Action," 113.

27. For "matters of concern," see Latour, "Why Has Critique Run Out of Steam?" For "matters of care," see Puig de la Bellacasa, *Matters of Care*.

28. See discussions in Gavin Brown et al., "Sedgwick's Geographies"; and Puig de la Bellacasa, "Matters of Care in Technoscience."

29. Hitt, *Bunch of Amateurs*.

30. Callon and Rabeharisoa, "Research 'in the Wild,'" 197.

31. Callon and Rabeharisoa, "Research 'in the Wild,'" 200.

32. Roelvink, "Collective Action," 117.

33. Cameron, Manhood, and Pomfrett, "Bodily Learning." On using this as a methodology, see Cameron, Gibson, and Hill, "Cultivating Hybrid Collectives."

34. See Dombroski, "Always Engaging"; Dombroski, "Hybrid Activist Collectives"; Dombroski, Healy, and McKinnon, "Care-Full Community Economies"; and Dombroski et al., "Journeying."

35. Massey, *For Space*, 151.

36. Tronto, "There Is an Alternative." See also Puig de la Bellacasa, *Matters of Care*, for a more-than-human perspective.

37. This argument is made in detail in Dombroski et al., "Journeying."

38. In recent years, I have seen many of these ideas circulate on Facebook under the growing no 'poo movement, so they may not seem particularly new. However, in 2008 and 2009, when these conversations were raging on the OzNappyfree off-topic forum, there was little public information available about the process of giving up shampoo, so these lessons had to be researched and learned by OzNappyfree members.

39. In fact, Transparency Market Research notes that in 2022, the dominant markets for shampoo bars are Australia, New Zealand, and China (www.transparency marketresearch.com/shampoo-bar-market.html), the three countries where this experimentation was undertaken in 2009. Of course, I have no evidence that it was because of OzNappyfree, but it does illustrate the degree to which the particularities of place play out in hygiene assemblages.

40. See van Eijk et al., "Menstrual Cup Use," which notes that support of peers is often needed to begin using menstrual cups.

41. I return here to the language used by Cameron, Gibson, and Hill, "Cultivating Hybrid Collectives."

42. Humans actually have a microbiome biodiversity crisis on our hands, with the biodiversity of gut and mouth bacteria becoming more homogeneous and reducing in diversity, with implications for human health. See Haahtela, "Biodiversity Hypothesis."

6. GUARDING LIFE

1. Roelvink, "Learning to Be Affected," 57.

2. Ruddick is careful to note that this thinking is available to all who do deep embodied nurturing work, but her starting point is mothers. Ruddick, *Maternal Thinking*.

3. Benjamin, *Viral Justice*.

4. Stephen Healy, in "Saint Francis," explores the interconnections between radical movements in our times of climate crisis and the radical early monastic "explosion" of the eleventh and twelfth centuries.

5. As discussed earlier, the Great Singularity refers to an imagination of the world critiques by postdevelopment theorists Boaventura de Sousa Santos and Arturo Escobar. I am sometimes tempted to call it the Great White Singularity.

6. To return to the opening quotes from Plumwood, "Ethics for Decolonisation," 1.

7. This is a point of which the late Julie Graham (of J. K. Gibson-Graham) often reminded us, in many different contexts.

Bibliography

Adams, Vincanne, Suellen Miller, Jennifer Chertow, Sienna Craig, Arlene Samen, and Michael Varner. "Having a 'Safe Delivery': Conflicting Views from Tibet." *Health Care for Women International* 26, no. 9 (2005): 821–51. doi.org/10.1080/07399330500 230920.

Anderson, Rosalind C., and Julius H. Anderson. "Acute Respiratory Effects of Diaper Emissions." *Archives of Environmental Health* 54, no. 5 (1999): 353–58.

Ashenburg, Katherine. *The Dirt on Clean: An Unsanitized History.* Toronto: Knopf Canada, 2007.

Attané, Isabelle. "'Trois enfants pour tous en Chine?" *Population et sociétés* 596 (2022): 1–4. doi.org/10.3917/popsoc.596.0001.

Aumônier, Simon, Michael Collins, and Peter Garrett. *An Update Lifecycle Assessment Study for Disposable and Reusable Nappies.* Bristol: Environment Agency, 2008.

Axel, Nick, Nikolaus Hirsch, and Troy Conrad Therrien. "Editorial—Survivance." *E-Flux Architecture,* May 2021. www.e-flux.com/architecture/survivance/393914/editorial-survivance.

Bai, Yana, Ning Cheng, Cipeng Jiang, Qi Wang, and Darueng Cao. "Survey on Cystic Echinococcosis in Tibetans, West China." *Acta Tropica* 82 (2002): 381–85. doi.org/10.1016/S0001-706X(02)00038-4.

Bakker, E., J. D. van Gool, and J. J. Wyndaele. "Results of a Questionnaire Evaluating Different Aspects of Personal and Familial Situation, and the Methods of Potty-Training in Two Groups of Children with a Different Outcome of Bladder Control." *Scandinavian Journal of Urology and Nephrology* 35 (2001): 370–76. doi.org/10.1080/003655901753224422.

Bakker, E., and J. J. Wyndaele. "Changes in the Toilet Training of Children during the Last 60 Years: The Cause of an Increase in Lower Urinary Tract Dysfunction?" *BJU International* 86, no. 3 (2000): 248–52. doi.org/10.1046/j.1464-410x.2000.00737.x.

Bauer, Ingrid. *Diaper Free! The Gentle Wisdom of Natural Infant Hygiene.* Salt Spring Island, B.C., Canada: Natural Wisdom, 2001.

Bender, Jeffrey M., and Rosemary C. She. "Elimination Communication: Diaper-Free in America." *Pediatrics* 140, no. 1 (2017): e20170398. doi.org/10.1542/peds.2017 -0398.

Benjamin, Ruha. *Viral Justice: How We Grow the World We Want.* Princeton, N.J.: Princeton University Press, 2022.

Black, Maggie, and Ben Fawcett. *The Last Taboo: Opening the Door on the Global Sanitation Crisis.* London: Earthscan, 2008.

Bobel, Christina. "Bounded Liberation: A Focused Study of La Leche League International." *Gender and Society* 15, no. 1 (2001): 130–51. doi.org/10.1177/089124301015 001007.

Bobel, Christina. "When Good Enough Isn't: Mother Blame in the Continuum Concept." *Journal of the Association for Research on Mothering* 6, no. 2 (2004): 68–78.

Boucke, Laurie. *Infant Potty Training: A Gentle and Primeval Method Adapted to Modern Living.* Lafayette, Colo.: White-Boucke, 2002.

Brazelton, Mary Augusta. "Frontiers of Immunology: Medical Migrations to Yunnan, Vaccine Research, and Public Health during the War with Japan, 1937–1945." In *China and the Globalization of Biomedicine,* edited by David Luesink, William H. Schneider, and Zhang Daqing, 183–214. Rochester: University of Rochester Press, 2019.

Brown, Gavin, Kath Browne, Michael Brown, Gerda Roelvink, Michelle Carnegie, and Ben Anderson. "Sedgwick's Geographies: Touching Space." *Progress in Human Geography* 35, no. 1 (2011): 121–31. doi.org/10.1177/0309132510386253.

Buckley, Sarah J. *Gentle Birth, Gentle Mothering.* Brisbane: One Moon, 2005.

Butler, Judith. *Gender Trouble.* New York: Routledge, 1990.

Cairns, Kate. "The 'Organic Child' Ideal Holds Mothers to an Impossible Standard." *Aeon,* February 19, 2020. aeon.co/ideas/the-organic-child-ideal-holds-mothers-to -an-impossible-standard.

Cairns, Kate, Josée Johnston, and Norah MacKendrick. "Feeding the 'Organic Child': Mothering through Ethical Consumption." *Journal of Consumer Culture* 13, no. 2 (2013): 97–118. doi.org/10.1177/1469540513480162.

Callon, Michel, and Vololona Rabeharisoa. "Research 'in the Wild' and the Shaping of New Social Identities." *Technology in Society* 25 (2003): 193–204. doi.org/10.1016/ S0160-791X(03)00021-6.

Cameron, Jenny. "On Experimentation." In *Manifesto for Living in the Anthropocene,* edited by Katherine Gibson, Deborah Bird Rose, and Ruth Fincher, 99–102. New York: Punctum, 2015.

Cameron, Jenny, Katherine Gibson, and Ann Hill. "Cultivating Hybrid Collectives: Research Methods for Enacting Community Food Economies in Australia and the Philippines." *Local Environment* 19, no. 1 (2014): 118–32. doi.org/10.1080/13549839.2013 .855892.

Cameron, Jenny, Craig Manhood, and Jamie Pomfrett. "Bodily Learning for a (Climate) Changing World: Registering Differences through Performative and Collective Research." *Local Environment* 16, no. 6 (2011): 493–508. doi.org/10.1080/1354983 9.2011.573473.

Campkin, Ben, and Rosie Cox, eds. *Dirt: New Geographies of Cleanliness and Contamination.* London: Bloomsbury, 2012.

Chen, Xinyin, and Leora C. Swartzman. "Health Beliefs and Experiences in Asian Cultures." In *Handbook of Cultural Health Psychology,* edited by Shahé S. Kazarian and David R. Evans, 389–410. San Diego, Calif.: Academic, 2001.

Cheng, Fung-Kei. "*Taijiao:* A Traditional Chinese Approach to Enhancing Fetal Growth through Maternal Physical and Mental Health." *Chinese Nursing Research* 3, no. 2 (2016): 49–53. doi.org/10.1016/j.cnre.2016.06.001.

Christie, Anna. "Toilet Training of Infants and Children in Australia: 2010 Parental Attitudes and Practices." Restraint Project, University of New South Wales, Sydney, 2012. https://web.maths.unsw.edu.au/~jim/annachristierpt10.pdf.

Chung, Yuehtsen Juliette. "Better Science and Better Race? Social Darwinism and Chinese Eugenics." *Isis* 105, no. 4 (2014): 793–802. doi.org/10.1086/679426.

Clarke, Adele E., Janet K. Shim, Laura Mamo, Jennifer Ruth Fosket, and Jennifer R. Fishman, eds. "Biomedicalization: A Theoretical and Substantive Introduction." In *Biomedicalization: Technoscience, Health, and Illness in the U.S.,* edited by Adele E. Clarke, Janet K. Shim, Laura Mamo, Jennifer Ruth Fosket, and Jennifer R. Fishman, 1–46. Durham, N.C.: Duke University Press, 2010.

Committee on Obstetric Practice. "Committee Opinion No. 543: Timing of Umbilical Cord Clamping after Birth." *Obstetrics and Gynecology* 120, no. 6 (2012): 1522–26.

Curtis, Valerie, and Adam Biran. "Dirt, Disgust, and Disease: Is Hygiene in Our Genes?" *Perspectives in Biology and Medicine* 44 (2001): 17–31. doi.org/10.1353/pbm .2001.0001.

Dashtdar, Mehrab, Mohammad Reza Dashtdar, Babak Dashtdar, Karima Kardi, and Mohammad Khabaz Shirazi. "The Concept of Wind in Traditional Chinese Medicine." *Journal of Pharmacopuncture* 19, no. 4 (2016): 293–302. doi.org/10.3831/kpi.2016 .19.030.

Das, Lina. "Mayim Bialik: How the *Big Bang Theory* Transformed Her Slow-Burning Career." *Stuff,* August 6, 2017. www.stuff.co.nz.

de Sousa Santos, Boaventura. "The WSF: Toward a Counter-hegemonic Globalization." In *World Social Forum: Challenging Empires,* edited by Jai Sen, Anita Anand, Arturo Escobar, and Peter Waterman, 235–45. New Delhi: Viveka Foundation, 2004.

deVries, Marten, and Rachel deVries. "Cultural Relativity of Toilet Training Readiness: A Perspective from East Africa." *Pediatrics* 60 (1977): 170–77. doi.org/10.1542/ peds.60.2.170.

"Diaper Rash May Be Due to Colored Dyes in Diapers." *Child Health Alert* 23 (2005): 3.

Dinerstein, Ana Cecilia, and Séverine Deneulin. "Hope Movements: Naming Mobilization in a Post-development World." *Development and Change* 43, no. 2 (2012): 584–602. doi.org/10.1111/j.1467-7660.2012.01765.x.

Dixon, Lesley, Joan Skinner, and Maralyn Foureur. "The Emotional and Hormonal Pathways of Labour and Birth: Integrating Mind, Body and Behaviour." *New Zealand College of Midwives Journal* 48 (2013): 15–23. hdl.handle.net/10453/31887.

Dombroski, Kelly. "Always Engaging with Others: Assembling an Antipodean, Hybrid Economic Geography Collective." *Dialogues in Human Geography* 3, no. 2 (2013): 217–21. doi.org/10.1177/2043820613493155.

Dombroski, Kelly. "Hybrid Activist Collectives: Reframing Mothers' Environmental and Caring Labour." *International Journal of Sociology and Social Policy* 36, no. 9/10 (2016): 629–46. doi.org/10.1108/ijssp-12-2015-0150.

Dombroski, Kelly. "Learning to Be Affected: Maternal Connection, Intuition and 'Elimination Communication.'" *Emotion, Space, and Society* 26 (2018): 72–79. doi.org/10.1016/j.emospa.2017.09.004.

Dombroski, Kelly. "Multiplying Possibilities: A Postdevelopment Approach to Hygiene and Sanitation in Northwest China." *Asia Pacific Viewpoint* 56, no. 3 (2015): 321–34. doi.org/10.1111/apv.12078.

Dombroski, Kelly. "Seeing Diversity, Multiplying Possibility: My Journey from Post-feminism to Postdevelopment with J. K. Gibson-Graham." In *The Palgrave Handbook of Gender and Development,* edited by Wendy Harcourt, 312–28. Basingstoke: Palgrave Macmillan, 2016.

Dombroski, Kelly. "What Other Countries Can Teach Us about Ditching Disposable Nappies." *The Conversation,* July 5, 2019. theconversation.com.

Dombroski, Kelly, Gradon Diprose, and Irene Boles. "Can the Commons Be Temporary? The Role of Transitional Commoning in Post-quake Christchurch." *Local Environment* 24, no. 4 (2019): 313–28. doi.org/10.1080/13549839.2019.1567480.

Dombroski, Kelly, Caihuan Duojie, and Katharine McKinnon. "Surviving Well: From Diverse Economies to Community Economies in Asia-Pacific." *Asia Pacific Viewpoint* 63, no. 1 (2022): 5–11. doi.org/10.1111/apv.12337.

Dombroski, Kelly, Stephen Healy, and Katharine McKinnon. "Care-Full Community Economies." In *Feminist Political Ecology and the Economics of Care,* edited by Wendy Harcourt and Christine Bauhardt, 99–115. London: Routledge, 2019.

Dombroski, Kelly, Katharine McKinnon, and Stephen Healy. "Beyond the Birth Wars: Diverse Assemblages of Care." *New Zealand Geographer* 72, no. 3 (2016): 230–39. doi.org/10.1111/nzg.12142.

Dombroski, Kelly, Hugh Nicholson, Rachael Shiels, Hannah Watkinson, and Amanda Yates. *Huritanga: 10 Years of Transformative Place-Making.* Ōtautahi, Christchurch: Life in Vacant Spaces, 2022.

Dombroski, Kelly, Alison Watkins, Helen Fitt, et al. "Journeying from 'I' to 'We': Assembling Hybrid Caring Collectives of Geography Doctoral Scholars." *Journal of Geography in Higher Education* 42, no. 1 (2018): 80–93. doi.org/10.1080/03098265.2017.1335295.

Dombroski, Kelly, and Amanda Yates. "The City as Laboratory: What Post-quake Christchurch Is Teaching Us about Urban Recovery and Transformation." *The Conversation,* September 19, 2022. theconversation.com.

Douglas, Mary. *Purity and Danger: An Analysis of Concepts of Pollution and Taboo.* London: Routledge, 2003.

Duong, Thi Hoa, Ulla-Britt Jansson, and Anna-Lena Hellström. "Vietnamese Mothers' Experiences with Potty Training Procedure for Children from Birth to 2 Years of

Age." *Journal of Pediatric Urology* 9, no. 6 (2013): 808–14. doi.org/10.1016/j.jpurol
.2012.10.023.

Duong, Thi Hoa, Ulla-Britt Jansson, Gundela Holmdahl, Ulla Sillén, and Anna-Lena
Hellström. "Urinary Bladder Control during the First 3 Years of Life in Healthy
Children in Vietnam—A Comparison Study with Swedish Children." *Journal of
Pediatric Urology* 9, no. 6 (2013): 700–706. doi.org/10.1016/j.jpurol.2013.04.022.

Dunn, Emily. "The Nappywars: When to Toilet Train?" *Sydney Morning Herald,* June 9,
2011.

Ehrenfeld, John R., and Andrew J. Hoffman. *Flourishing: A Frank Conversation about
Sustainability.* London: Routledge, 2013.

Ekinsmyth, Carol. "Challenging the Boundaries of Entrepreneurship: The Spatialities and Practices of U.K. 'Mumpreneurs.'" *Geoforum* 42, no. 1 (2011): 104–14. doi
.org/10.1016/j.geoforum.2010.10.005.

Escobar, Arturo. "Beyond the Third World: Imperial Globality, Global Coloniality
and Anti-globalisation Social Movements." *Third World Quarterly* 25, no. 1 (2004):
207–30. doi.org/10.1080/0143659042000185417.

Escobar, Arturo. *Designs for the Pluriverse: Radical Interdependence, Autonomy, and the
Making of Worlds.* Durham, N.C.: Duke University Press, 2018.

Escobar, Arturo. "Development, Violence, and the New Imperial Order." *Development* 47, no. 1 (2004): 15–21. doi.org/10.1057/palgrave.development.1100014.

Escobar, Arturo, and Wendy Harcourt. "Post-development Possibilities: A Conversation." *Development* 61, no. 1 (2018): 6–8. doi.org/10.1057/s41301-018-0184-3.

Escobar, Arturo, and Ho-Won Jeong. "Postdevelopment: Beyond the Critique of
Development." In *The New Agenda for Peace Research,* edited by Ho-Won Jeong,
223–32. London: Routledge, 2019.

Esteva, Gustavo. "Development." In *The Development Dictionary,* edited by W. Sachs.
London: Zed, 1992.

Esteva, Gustavo, and Arturo Escobar. "Post-development @ 25: On 'Being Stuck' and
Moving Forward, Sideways, Backward and Otherwise." *Third World Quarterly* 38,
no. 12 (2017): 2559–72. doi.org/10.1080/01436597.2017.1334545.

Farquhar, Judith. *A Way of Life: Things, Thought, and Action in Chinese Medicine.* New
Haven, Conn.: Yale University Press, 2020.

Farquhar, Judith, and Lili Lai. *Gathering Medicines: Nation and Knowledge in China's
Mountain South.* Chicago: University of Chicago Press, 2021.

Feng, Emily. "China Is Removing Domes from Mosques as Part of a Push to Make
Them More 'Chinese.'" NPR, October 24, 2021. www.npr.org.

Flaws, Bob. *A Handbook of TCM Pediatrics: A Practitioner's Guide to the Care and Treatment of Common Childhood Diseases.* Boulder, Colo.: Blue Poppy, 1997.

Fox, Haylee, Stephanie M. Topp, Daniel Lindsay, and Emily Callander. "Response to:
The 'Cascade of Interventions': Does It Really Exist?" *Birth* 49, no. 2 (2022): 173–74.

Frazier, Mya. "How P&G Brought the Diaper Revolution to China." CBS News,
January 11, 2010. www.cbsnews.com.

Gibson-Graham, J. K. *A Postcapitalist Politics.* Minneapolis: University of Minnesota
Press, 2006.

Gibson-Graham, J. K. "Reading for Economic Difference." In *The Handbook of Diverse Economies*, edited by J. K. Gibson-Graham and K. Dombroski, 476–87. Cheltenham, England, U.K.: Edward Elgar, 2020.

Gibson-Graham, J. K. "Surplus Possibilities: Postdevelopment and Community Economies." *Singapore Journal of Tropical Geography* 26, no. 1 (2005): 4–26.

Gibson-Graham, J. K., Jenny Cameron, and Stephen Healy. *Take Back the Economy: An Ethical Guide for Transforming Our Communities*. Minneapolis: University of Minnesota Press, 2013.

Gibson, Katherine, Deborah Bird Rose, and Ruth Fincher, eds. *Manifesto for Living in the Anthropocene*. New York: Punctum, 2015.

Global Public–Private Partnership for Handwashing. *The Handwashing Handbook: A Guide for Developing a Hygiene Promotion Program to Increase Handwashing with Soap.* 2015. globalhandwashing.org/wp-content/uploads/2015/03/Handwashing_Handbook_web-1.pdf.

Green, Alexander, J. Emilio Carrillo, and Joseph Betancourt. "Why the Disease-Based Model of Medicine Fails Our Patients." *Western Journal of Medicine* 176, no. 2 (2002): 141–43.

Grosz, Elizabeth. *Volatile Bodies: Toward a Corporeal Feminism*. St. Leonards, New South Wales, Australia: Allen & Unwin, 1994.

Haahtela, Tari. "A Biodiversity Hypothesis." *Allergy* 74, no. 8 (2019): 1445–56. doi.org/10.1111/all.13763.

Hammerstrom, Erik. "A Buddhist Critique of Scientism." *Journal of Chinese Buddhist Studies* 27 (2014): 35–57.

Haraway, Donna. "Situated Knowledges: The Science Question in Feminism and the Privilege of Partial Perspective." *Feminist Studies* 14, no. 3 (1988): 575–99. doi.org/10.2307/3178066.

Harcourt, Wendy. *Body Politics in Development: Critical Debates in Gender and Development*. London: Bloomsbury, 2009.

Hashemi, Shervin. "Sanitation Sustainability Index: A Pilot Approach to Develop a Community-Based Indicator for Evaluating Sustainability of Sanitation Systems." *Sustainability* 12, no. 17 (2020): 6937. doi.org/10.3390/su12176937.

Healy, Stephen. "Saint Francis in Climate-Changing Times: Form of Life, the Highest Poverty, and Postcapitalist Politics." *Rethinking Marxism* 28, no. 3–4 (2016): 367–84. doi.org/10.1080/08935696.2016.1243422.

Hechler, Christine, Roseriet Beijers, J. Marianne Riksen-Walraven, and Carolina de Weerth. "Are Cortisol Concentrations in Human Breast Milk Associated with Infant Crying?" *Developmental Psychobiology* 60, no. 6 (2018): 639–50. doi.org/10.1002/dev.21761.

Hitt, Jack. *Bunch of Amateurs: A Search for the American Character*. New York: Crown, 2012.

Hong, Fan. *Footbinding, Feminism, and Freedom: The Liberation of Women's Bodies in Modern China*. New York: Frank Cass, 1997.

Hopgood, Mei-Ling. *How Eskimos Keep Their Babies Warm: And Other Adventures in Parenting (from Argentina to Tanzania and Everywhere in Between)*. New York: Algonquin, 2012.

Hsu, Elisabeth. "The History of Chinese Medicine in the People's Republic of China and Its Globalization." *East Asian Science, Technology, and Society* 2, no. 4 (2008): 465–84. doi.org/10.1215/s12280-009-9072-y.

Iossifova, Deljana. "Everyday Practices of Sanitation under Uneven Urban Development in Contemporary Shanghai." *Environment and Urbanization* 27, no. 2 (2015): 541–54. doi.org/10.1177/0956247815581748.

Iossifova, Deljana. "Urban (Sanitation) Transformation in China: A Toilet Revolution and Its Socio-eco-technical Entanglements." In *Urban Transformations and Public Health in the Emergent City*, edited by M. Keith and A. de Sousa Santos, 102–22. Manchester, England, U.K.: Manchester University Press, 2020.

Jewitt, Sarah. "Geographies of Shit: Spatial and Temporal Variations in Attitudes towards Human Waste." *Progress in Human Geography* 35, no. 5 (2011): 608–26. doi.org/10.1177/0309132510394704.

Karasik, Lana B., Catherine S. Tamis-LeMonda, Ori Ossmy, and Karen E. Adolph. "The Ties that Bind: Cradling in Tajikistan." *PLoS One* 13, no. 10 (2018): e0204428. doi.org/10.1371/journal.pone.0204428.

Kaul, Shivani, Bengi Akbulut, Federico Demaria, and Julien-François Gerber. "Alternatives to Sustainable Development: What Can We Learn from the Pluriverse in Practice?" *Sustainability Science* 17, no. 4 (2022): 1149–58. doi.org/10.1007/s11625-022-01210-2.

Kedgely, Sue. *Mum's the Word: The Untold Story of Motherhood in New Zealand.* Auckland: Random House, 1996.

Klein, Elise, and Carlos Eduardo Morreo. *Postdevelopment in Practice: Alternatives, Economies, Ontologies.* New York: Routledge, 2019.

Kothari, Uma. "From Colonialism to Development: Reflections of Former Colonial Officers." *Commonwealth and Comparative Politics* 44, no. 1 (2006): 118–36. doi.org/10.1080/14662040600624502.

Kothari, Ashish, Ariel Salleh, Arturo Escobar, Federico Demaria, and Alberto Acosta, eds. *Pluriverse: A Post-development Dictionary.* New York: Columbia University Press, 2019.

Kristeva, Julia. *Powers of Horror: An Essay on Abjection.* Translated by Leon S. Roudiez. New York: Columbia University Press, 1982.

Lahiri-Dutt, Kuntala. "Medicalising Menstruation: A Feminist Critique of the Political Economy of Menstrual Hygiene Management in South Asia." *Gender, Place, and Culture* 22, no. 8 (2015): 1158–76. doi.org/10.1080/0966369x.2014.939156.

Largo, R. H., L. Molinari, K. von Siebenthal, and U. Wolfensberger. "Development of Bladder and Bowel Control: Significance of Prematurity, Perinatal Risk Factors, Psychomotor Development and Gender." *European Journal of Pediatrics* 158 (1999): 115–22. doi.org/10.1007/s004310051030.

Larsen, Soren C., and Jay T. Johnson. *Being Together in Place: Indigenous Coexistence in a More Than Human World.* Minneapolis: University of Minnesota Press, 2017.

Latour, Bruno. "How to Talk about the Body? The Normative Dimension of Science Studies." *Body and Society* 10 (2004): 205–29. doi.org/10.1177/1357034X04042943.

Latour, Bruno. "Why Has Critique Run Out of Steam? From Matters of Fact to Matters of Concern." *Critical Inquiry* 30 (2004): 225–48.

Latour, Bruno, and Steve Woolgar. *Laboratory Life: The Construction of Scientific Facts.* Princeton, N.J.: Princeton University Press, 1986.

Law, John. *After Method: Mess in Social Science Research.* London: Routledge, 2004.

Law, John. "What's Wrong with a One-World World?" *Distinktion: Scandinavian Journal of Social Theory* 16, no. 1 (2015): 126–39. doi.org/10.1080/1600910X.2015.1020066.

Lei, Sean Hsiang-lin. "Habituating Individuality: The Framing of Tuberculosis and Its Material Solutions in Republican China." *Bulletin of the History of Medicine* 84 (2010): 248–79.

Lei, Sean Hsiang-lin. "Moral Community of *Weisheng*: Contesting Hygiene in Republican China." *East Asian Science, Technology, and Society* 3, no. 4 (2009): 475–504. doi.org/10.1215/s12280-009-9109-2.

Lei, Sean Hsiang-lin. *Neither Donkey nor Horse: Medicine in the Struggle over China's Modernity.* Chicago: University of Chicago Press, 2014.

Lei, Sean Hsiang-lin. "Sovereignty and the Microscope." In *Health and Hygiene in Chinese East Asia: Policies and Publics in the Long Twentieth Century,* edited by Angela Ki Che Leung and Charlotte Furth, 79–108. Durham, N.C.: Duke University Press, 2010.

Leung, Angela Ki Che. "The Evolution of the Idea of *Chuanran* Contagion in Imperial China." In *Health and Hygiene in Chinese East Asia: Policies and Publics in the Long Twentieth Century,* edited by Angela Ki Che Leung and Charlotte Furth, 25–49. Durham, N.C.: Duke University Press, 2010.

Leung, Angela Ki Che, and Charlotte Furth, eds. *Health and Hygiene in Chinese East Asia: Policies and Publics in the Long Twentieth Century.* Durham, N.C.: Duke University Press, 2010.

Li, Tiaoying, Xingwang Chen, Ren Zhen, et al. "Widespread Co-endemicity of Human Cystic and Alveolar Echinococcosis on the Eastern Tibetan Plateau, Northwest Sichuan/Southeast Qinghai, China." *Acta Tropica* 113, no. 3 (2010): 248–56. doi.org/10.1016/j.actatropica.2009.11.006.

Liedloff, Jean. *The Continuum Concept.* Boulder, Colo.: Perseus, 1986.

Liu, Qi, Alison L. Browne, and Deljana Iossifova. "A Socio-material Approach to Resource Consumption and Environmental Sustainability of Tourist Accommodations in a Chinese Hot Spring Town." *Sustainable Production and Consumption* 30 (2022): 424–37. doi.org/10.1016/j.spc.2021.12.021.

Liu, Xianchen, Zhenxiao Sun, Makoto Uchiyama, Y. A. N. Li, and Masako Okawa. "Attaining Nocturnal Urinary Control, Nocturnal Enuresis, and Behavioral Problems in Chinese Children Aged 6 through 16 Years." *Journal of the American Academy of Child and Adolescent Psychiatry* 39, no. 12 (2000): 1557–64. doi.org/10.1097/00004583-200012000-00020.

Liu, Xin. *The Mirage of China: Anti-humanism, Narcissism, and Corporeality of the Contemporary World.* New York: Berghahn, 2009.

Liu, Xin. *The Otherness of Self: A Genealogy of the Self in Contemporary China.* Ann Arbor: University of Michigan Press, 2002.

Longhurst, R. *Bodies: Exploring Fluid Boundaries.* London: Routledge, 2001.

Longhurst, R. "(Dis)embodied Geographies." *Progress in Human Geography* 21, no. 4 (1997): 486–501.

Luesink, David. "Introduction: China and the Globalization of Biomedicine." In *China and the Globalization of Biomedicine,* edited by David Luesink, William H. Schneider, and Zhang Daqing, 1–34. Rochester: University of Rochester Press, 2019.

Lynteris, Christos. "Plague Masks: The Visual Emergence of Anti-epidemic Personal Protection Equipment." *Medical Anthropology* 37, no. 6 (2018): 442–57. doi.org/10.1080/01459740.2017.1423072.

Massey, Doreen. *For Space.* Los Angeles: Sage, 2005.

McGregor, Andrew. "New Possibilities? Shifts in Postdevelopment Theory and Practice." *Geography Compass* 3 (2009): 1688–702. doi.org/10.1111/j.1749-8198.2009.00260.x.

McKinnon, Katharine. *Birthing Work: The Collective Labour of Childbirth.* Singapore: Palgrave Macmillan, 2020.

McKinnon, Katharine. "The Geopolitics of Birth." *Area* 48, no. 3 (2016): 285–91. doi.org/10.1111/area.12131.

McKinnon, Katharine, Stephen Healy, and Kelly Dombroski. "Surviving Well Together: Postdevelopment, Maternity Care, and the Politics of Ontological Pluralism." In *Postdevelopment in Practice: Alternatives, Economies, Ontologies,* edited by Elise Klein and Carlos Eduardo Morreo, 190–202. London: Routledge, 2019.

Men, Jiuzhang, and Lei Guo. *A General Introduction to Traditional Chinese Medicine.* Boca Raton, Fla.: CRC Press, 2010.

Minchin, M. "Infant Formula: A Mass, Uncontrolled Trial in Perinatal Care." *Birth* 14 (1987): 25–34. doi.org/10.1111/j.1523-536X.1987.tb01445.x.

Mol, Annemarie. *The Body Multiple: Ontology in Medical Practice.* Durham, N.C.: Duke University Press, 2003.

Mothering. "The Politics of Diapers: A Timeline." 2003. www.mothering.com/threads/the-politics-of-diapers-a-timeline.1622389.

Narain, Jaya. "Mother, 25, Reunited with Two Children Eight Months after They Were Taken into Care When a Burst Nappy Horribly Scalded Young Daughter's Leg." *Daily Mail,* updated July 17, 2012. www.dailymail.co.uk.

"'Not a Joke': Mums Floored by Potty-Trained Baby on TikTok." *New Zealand Herald,* January 14, 2022. www.nzherald.co.nz.

Notten, Philippa, Alexandra Gower, and Yvonne Lewis. "Single-Use Nappies and Their Alternatives: Recommendations from Life Cycle Assessments." United Nations Environment Program, March 2021. www.lifecycleinitiative.org.

O'Brien, Kate, Rachel Olive, Yu-Chieh Hsu, Luke Morris, Richard Bell, and Nick Kendall. "Life Cycle Assessment: Reusable and Disposable Nappies in Australia." University of Queensland School of Engineering, Brisbane, 2009. www.parliament.act.gov.au/__data/assets/pdf_file/0006/2096268/08.1-Attachment-Life-Cycle-Assessment-Reusable-and-Disposable-Nappies.pdf.

Olson, Andrea. *Go Diaper Free: A Simple Handbook for Elimination Communication.* Asheville, N.C.: Tiny World, 2021.

Paddison, Laura. "Reuse? Compost? Dump? Solving the Eco-conundrum of Nappies." *Guardian,* November 20, 2021. www.theguardian.com.

Pillsbury, Barbara L. K. "'Doing the Month': Confinement and Convalescence of Chinese Women after Childbirth." *Social Science and Medicine* 12 (1978): 11–22. doi .org/10.1016/0160-7987(78)90003-0.

Płotka-Wasylka, Justyna, Patrycja Makoś-Chełstowska, Aleksandra Kurowska-Susdorf, et al. "End-of-Life Management of Single-Use Baby Diapers: Analysis of Technical, Health and Environment Aspects." *Science of the Total Environment* 836 (2022): 155339. doi.org/10.1016/j.scitotenv.2022.155339.

Plumwood, Val. *Environmental Culture: The Ecological Crisis of Reason.* New York: Routledge, 2002.

Plumwood, Val. "A Review of Deborah Bird Rose's *Reports from a Wild Country: Ethics for Decolonisation.*" *Australian Humanities Review,* August 1, 2007. australianhuman itiesreview.org.

Puig de la Bellacasa, María. "Matters of Care in Technoscience: Assembling Neglected Things." *Social Studies of Science* 41, no. 1 (2011): 85–106. doi.org/10.1177/03063127103 80301.

Puig de la Bellacasa, María. *Matters of Care: Speculative Ethics in More Than Human Worlds.* Minneapolis: University of Minnesota Press, 2017.

Ramaswamy, Chitra. "The Parents Toilet-Training Their Newborn Babies: 'You Get Instant Feedback.'" *Guardian,* June 26, 2017. www.theguardian.com.

Robinson, Lena. *Cross-Cultural Child Development for Social Workers: An Introduction.* London: Bloomsbury, 2020.

Roelvink, Gerda. *Building Dignified Worlds: Geographies of Collective Action.* Minneapolis: University of Minnesota Press, 2016.

Roelvink, Gerda. "Collective Action and the Politics of Affect." *Emotion, Space, and Society* 3, no. 2 (2010): 111–18. doi.org/10.1016/j.emospa.2009.10.004.

Roelvink, Gerda. "Learning to Be Affected by Earth Others." In *Manifesto for Living in the Anthropocene,* edited by K. Gibson, Deborah Bird Rose, and Ruth Fincher, 57–62. Brooklyn: Punctum, 2015.

Roelvink, Gerda, Kevin St. Martin, and J. K. Gibson-Graham, eds. *Making Other Worlds Possible: Performing Diverse Economies.* Minneapolis: University of Minnesota Press, 2015.

Rogaski, Ruth. *Hygienic Modernity: Meanings of Health and Disease in Treaty-Port China.* Berkeley: University of California Press, 2004.

Rogoff, Barbara. *The Cultural Nature of Human Development.* Oxford: Oxford University Press, 2003.

Rudan, Igor, Kit Yee Chan, Jian S. F. Zhang, et al. "Causes of Deaths in Children Younger than 5 Years in China in 2008." *Lancet* 375, no. 9720 (2010): 1083–89. doi .org/10.1016/S0140-6736(10)60060-8.

Ruddick, Sara. *Maternal Thinking: Towards a Politics of Peace.* London: Women's Press, 1989.

Schafer, Robyn, and Julia C. Phillippi. "Group B Streptococcal Bacteriuria in Pregnancy: An Evidence-Based, Patient-Centered Approach to Care." *Journal of Midwifery and Women's Health* 65, no. 3 (2020): 376–81. doi.org/10.1111/jmwh.13085.

Scholars Concerned for Life in the Anthropocene. *Manifesto for Living in the Anthropocene*. New York: Punctum, 2015.

Schum, Timothy R., Thomas M. Kolb, Timothy L. McAuliffe, Mark D. Simms, Richard L. Underhill, and Marla Lewis. "Sequential Acquisition of Toilet-Training Skills: A Descriptive Study of Gender and Age Differences in Normal Children." *Pediatrics* 109, no. 3 (2002): e48. doi.org/10.1542/peds.109.3.e48.

Sears, William, and Martha Sears. *The Attachment Parenting Book: A Commonsense Guide to Understanding and Nurturing Your Baby*. Boston: Little, Brown, 2001.

Sedgwick, Eve Kosofosky. *Tendencies*. London: Routledge, 1993.

Shih, Shu-mei. *The Lure of the Modern: Writing Modernism in Semicolonial China, 1917–1937*. Berkeley: University of California Press, 2001.

Shove, Elizabeth. *Comfort, Cleanliness, and Convenience: The Social Organization of Normality*. Oxford: Berg, 2003.

Shove, Elizabeth. "Social Theory and Climate Change." *Theory, Culture, and Society* 27, no. 2–3 (2010): 277–88. doi.org/10.1177/0263276410361498.

Sibonney, Claire. "Elimination Communication: Can Infants Actually Be Potty Trained?" *Today's Parent,* May 24, 2019.

Sillén, Ulla. "Bladder Function in Healthy Neonates and Its Development during Infancy." *Journal of Urology* 166, no. 6 (2001): 2376–81. doi.org/10.1016/S0022-5347(05)65594-2.

Smith, Virginia S. *Clean: A History of Personal Hygiene and Purity*. Oxford: Oxford University Press, 2007.

Snowden, Frank M. *Epidemics and Society: From the Black Death to the Present*. New Haven, Conn.: Yale University Press, 2019.

Strand, Mark A., Judith Perry, Jinzhi Guo, Jinping Zhao, and Craig Janes. "Doing the Month: Rickets and Post-partum Convalesence in Rural China." *Midwifery* 25 (2009): 588–96. doi.org/10.1016/j.midw.2007.10.008.

Sun, Min, and Simone Rugolotto. "Assisted Infant Toilet Training in a Western Family Setting." *Journal of Developmental and Behavioral Pediatrics* 25, no. 2 (2004): 99–101. doi.org/10.1097/00004703-200404000-00004.

Sun, Shangyang. "The Apostate Nie Yuntai's Comparison between Christianity and Buddhism and Its Inspiration to Sino-Christian Theology." *Logos and Pneuma: Chinese Journal of Theology,* no. 33 (2010): 145–76.

Tan, Kevin Y. L. "The Plague Fighter: Dr. Wu Lien-Teh and His Work." *Biblioasia,* July–September 2020, 16–23. biblioasia.nlb.gov.sg/vol-16/issue-2/jul-sep-2020/plague/.

Thomassen, Bjørn. "Anthropology and Its Many Modernities: When Concepts Matter." *Journal of the Royal Anthropological Institute* 18, no. 1 (2012): 160–78. doi.org/10.1111/j.1467-9655.2011.01736.x.

Todd, Zoe. "An Indigenous Feminist's Take on the Ontological Turn: 'Ontology' Is Just Another Word for Colonialism." *Journal of Historical Sociology* 29, no. 1 (2016): 4–22. doi.org/10.1111/johs.12124.

Tronto, Joan. "There Is an Alternative: *Homines Curans* and the Limits of Neoliberalism." *International Journal of Care and Caring* 1, no. 1 (2017): 27–43. doi.org/10.1332/239788217X14866281687583.

Tsing, Anna Lowenhaupt. *Friction: An Ethnography of Global Connection.* Princeton, N.J.: Princeton University Press, 2005.

Tsing, Anna Lowenhaupt. *In the Realm of the Diamond Queen.* Princeton, N.J.: Princeton University Press, 1993.

Tsing, Anna Lowenhaupt. *The Mushroom at the End of the World: On the Possibility of Life in Capitalist Ruins.* Princeton, N.J.: Princeton University Press, 2015.

Underhill-Sem, Yvonne. "Marked Bodies in Marginalized Places: Understanding Rationalities in Global Discourses." *Development* 46, no. 2 (2003): 13–17. doi.org/10.1057/palgrave.development.1110437.

van Eijk, Anna Maria, Garazi Zulaika, Madeline Lenchner, et al. "Menstrual Cup Use, Leakage, Acceptability, Safety, and Availability: A Systematic Review and Meta-analysis." *Lancet Public Health* 4, no. 8 (2019): e376–93. doi.org/10.1016/S2468-2667(19)30111-2.

Vandegrift, Roo, Ashley C. Bateman, Kyla N. Siemens, et al. "Cleanliness in Context: Reconciling Hygiene with a Modern Microbial Perspective." *Microbiome* 5, no. 1 (2017): 76. doi.org/10.1186/s40168-017-0294-2.

Veith, Ilza. "Introduction: Analysis of the *Huang Ti Nei Ching Su Wen.*" In *The Yellow Emperor's Classic of Internal Medicine,* 1–76. 1975; reprint, Oakland: University of California Press, 2016.

Vizenor, Gerald. *Native Liberty: Natural Reason and Cultural Survivance.* Lincoln: University of Nebraska Press, 2009.

Wang, Ying, Yanqun Liu, Jinbing Bai, and Xiaoli Chen. "The Effect of Maternal Postpartum Practices on Infant Gut Microbiota: A Chinese Cohort Study." *Microorganisms* 7, no. 11 (2019): 511. doi.org/10.3390/microorganisms7110511.

Wohl, Jessica. "P&G Faces Growing Backlash over Updated Pampers." Reuters, April 19, 2010. www.reuters.com/article/us-procter-pampers-idUSTRE63J03E20100420.

World Health Organization. "International Code of Marketing of Breast-Milk Substitutes." January 26, 1981. www.who.int/publications/i/item/9241541601.

Wu, Hsi-Yang. "Achieving Urinary Continence in Children." *Nature Reviews Urology* 7, no. 7 (2010): 371–77. doi.org/10.1038/nrurol.2010.78.

Wu, Hsi-Yang. "Can Evidence-Based Medicine Change Toilet-Training Practice?" *Arab Journal of Urology* 11, no. 1 (2013): 13–18. doi.org/10.1016/j.aju.2012.11.001.

Xu, Jianchu, Yong Yang, Nyima Tashi, Rita Sharma, and Jing Fang. "Understanding Land Use, Livelihoods, and Health Transitions among Tibetan Nomads: A Case from Gangga Township, Dingri County, Tibetan Autonomous Region of China." *Ecohealth* 5 (2008): 104–14. doi.org/10.1007/s10393-008-0173-1.

Xu, Sanchun, and Danian Hu. "Barefoot Doctors and the 'Health Care Revolution' in Rural China: A Study Centered on Shandong Province." *Endeavour* 41, no. 3 (2017): 136–45. doi.org/10.1016/j.endeavour.2017.06.004.

Yan, Wudan. "What Can and Can't Be Learned from a Doctor in China Who Pioneered Masks." *New York Times,* May 19, 2021. www.nytimes.com.

Yang, Shucai, Quanbao Jiang, and Jesús J. Sánchez-Barricarte. "China's Fertility Change: An Analysis with Multiple Measures." *Population Health Metrics* 20, no. 1 (2022): 12. doi.org/10.1186/s12963-022-00290-7.

Yang, Jui-sung. "From Discourse of Weakness to Discourse of Empowerment: The Topos of the 'Sick Man of East Asia' in Modern China." In *Discourses of Weakness in Modern China: Historical Diagnoses of the "Sick Man of East Asia,"* edited by Iwo Amelung, 25–78. Frankfurt: Campus Verlag, 2020.

Yates, Amanda, Kelly Dombroski, and Rita Dionisio. "Dialogues for Wellbeing in an Ecological Emergency: Wellbeing-led Governance Frameworks and Transformative Indigenous Tools." *Dialogues in Human Geography* 13, no. 2 (2023): 268–87. doi .org/10.1177/20438206221102957.

Yau, Elaine. "China Enraged by 'Sick Man of Asia' Headline, but Its Origin May Surprise Many." *South China Morning Post* (Hong Kong), February 27, 2020. www .scmp.com.

Yeung, C. K., M. L. Godley, C. K. W. Ho, et al. "Some New Insights into Bladder Function in Infancy." *British Journal of Urology* 76, no. 2 (1995): 235–40. doi.org/ 10.1111/j.1464-410X.1995.tb07682.x.

Youkee, Mat, and Emma Graham-Harrison. "'Miracle, Miracle': Lone Children Survive 40 Days in Amazon Jungle." *Guardian,* June 10, 2023. www.theguardian.com.

Yu, Sarah Xia. "Masks and Geopolitics in Richard Pearson Strong's Photos of the Manchurian Plague Epidemic, 1910–1911." *Harvard Library Bulletin,* 2021. dash.har vard.edu/bitstream/handle/1/37368736/HLB_2021_Yu.pdf.

Yu, Xinzhong. "The Treatment of Night Soil and Waste in Modern China." In *Health and Hygiene in Chinese East Asia: Policies and Publics in the Long Twentieth Century,* edited by Angela Ki Che Leung and Charlotte Furth, 51–72. Durham, N.C.: Duke University Press, 2010.

Zeng, Xinying, Tim Adair, Lijun Wang, et al. "Measuring the Completeness of Death Registration in 2844 Chinese Counties in 2018." *BMC Medicine* 18, no. 1 (2020): 176. doi.org/10.1186/s12916-020-01632-8.

Zhang Jingyue. *Complete Compendium of Zhang Jingyue.* Translated by Allen Tsaur. Edited by Michael Brown. 3 vols. New York: Purple Cloud Press, 2020.

Zheng, Ruoting, and Fangchao Fan. "Wealth Lies in Virtue: How to Preserve Wealth by Nie Yuntai and Its Relevance to Modern Society." *China Nonprofit Review* 4, no. 2 (2012): 275–84. doi.org/10.1163/18765149-12341249.

Index

Page numbers in *italics* refer to figures.

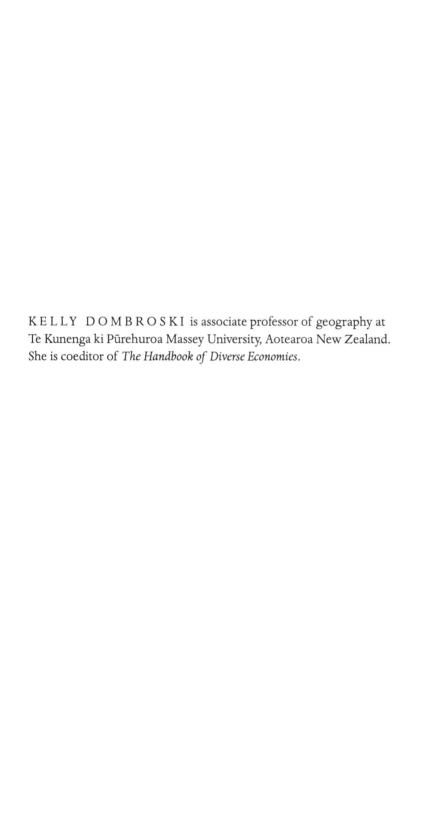

KELLY DOMBROSKI is associate professor of geography at Te Kunenga ki Pūrehuroa Massey University, Aotearoa New Zealand. She is coeditor of *The Handbook of Diverse Economies*.

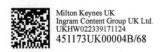

9 780816 679850